KETTLEBELL GUIDE FOR BEGINNERS
21-Days to Kettlebell Training

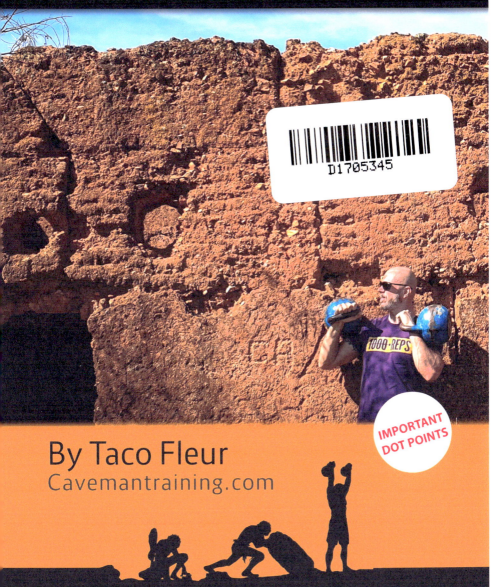

By Taco Fleur
Cavemantraining.com

IMPORTANT DOT POINTS

21-days to lay a solid foundation for kettlebells.

Kettlebell Guide for Beginners
21-Days to Kettlebell Training

This book is a quick introduction to kettlebell training for beginners. It's a kettlebell guide for beginners with dot points rather than lengthy explanations. This book is all about quick access to information. I've taken feedback from other books onboard where people said there was too much information and they just wanted to dive straight in. This book is also cheaper than other books as I've left links to additional videos out. I am including a bonus voucher code toward the end of the book which you can use to purchase a 2 hour streaming video which covers all the information from these 21 days step-by-step, it's fully optional to purchase and not required but a great additional for those who are more visual and like to hear someone talk.

Table of Contents

How to submit your assessment 6
Day 1 Warming up and priming for kettlebell training 7
Day 2 Stretching and mobility for kettlebell training 21
Day 3 Kettlebell anatomy and grip 33
Day 4 Safely lifting the kettlebell with a squat 35
Day 5 Safely lifting the kettlebell with a hip hinge 38
Day 6 Assisted kettlebell clean 41
Day 7 Kettlebell squat swing 48
Day 8 Kettlebell hip hinge swing 52
Day 9 Kettlebell pendulum swing 56
Day 10 Double arm swing clean 60
Day 11 Kettlebell dead clean 65
Day 12 Kettlebell swing clean 73
Day 13 Kettlebell racking 77
Day 14 Kettlebell pressing 80
Day 15 Kettlebell rowing 83
Day 16 Kettlebell American swing 86
Day 17 Double kettlebell dead swing clean 89
Day 18 Recap and additional kettlebell tips 93
Day 19 Kettlebell programming and goals 95
Day 20 Kettlebell workout 97
Day 21 Common kettlebell injuries and annoyances 100
VOUCHER CODES 101

About the Author

My name is Taco Fleur, and I'm an IKFF Certified Kettlebell Trainer, Russian Girevoy Sport Institute Kettlebell Coach, Kettlebell Level 1 + 2 Trainer, Kettlebell Science and Application, CrossFit Level 1 Trainer, MMA Conditioning Level 1, Kettlebell Sport IKMF Rank 2, MMA Fitness Level 1 + 2, Punchfit Trainer and Plyometrics Trainer Certified, with a purple belt in Brazilian Jiu-Jitsu. I have owned and set-up 3 functional kettlebell gyms in Australia and Vietnam, and lived in the Netherlands, Australia, Vietnam, and Thailand. I'm currently living in Spain.

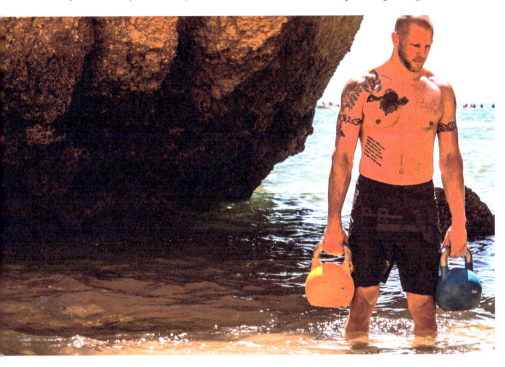

The first thing I'd like you to know about me is that I do **not** know everything, I don't pretend to know everything, and I never will. I'm on a path of life-long learning. I believe there is always something to learn from someone, no matter who they are. I've been physically active since the day I arrived on this earth in 1973. I got serious about training in 1999, touched a kettlebell for the first time in 2004, and got serious about kettlebell training in 2009. I'm here to do what I love most, and that is to share my knowledge with the world.

Some of my personal bests are 400 burpees performed in under one hour; 500 kettlebell snatches, 500 swings and 500 double-unders all completed in one session; 250 alternating dead clean and presses in one session with 20kg; 200 pull-ups in one session; 200 unbroken kettlebell swings with a 28kg; most kettlebell swings completed in one session with a 28kg (1,501); most total kettlebell swings done in 28 days with a 28kg (11,111); windmill with a 40kg kettlebell; lugged a kettlebell up a 1,184m mountain; 160kg dead lift; 250 alternating dead clean and presses in one session with 20kg; 100 snatches on sand with a 24kg kettlebell; 300 unbroken clean and jerk with 20kg/44lbs; 85kg Olympic Squat Snatch; Gold medalist with 30 minutes of unbroken 16kg half snatches for a total of 532 reps; and one of my favorites is lugging the first kettlebell up the highest mountain in mainland Spain 3,479m/11,414f with 16kg. I mention these PBs not to boast but to demonstrate that

I have a good understanding of technique and movement across different areas. This demonstrates especially with the high reps, an area in which most commonly tearing of the hands occurs.

My own training and goals are geared around GPP (General Physical Preparedness) which involves kettlebell training, calisthenics, and CrossFit. I like high-volume reps but also like greasing the groove now and again. My main goals are to remains as agile as possible, remain mobile, train in as many planes of movements as possible, and learn as many different exercise combinations and movements as possible while having fun and enjoying Brazilian Jiu Jitsu. I'm no Arnold Schwarzenegger and never will be, but strength is not solely defined by physical appearance and huge bulging muscles.

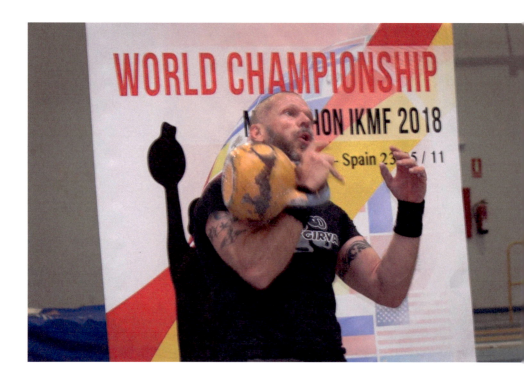

You can read more about my training, philosophy, and other ramblings on my website, www.cavemantraining.com, and on my YouTube channel, bit.ly/youtube-cavemantraining, which at the time of writing has over 34,000 subscribers and more than 6 million views.

SUBSCRIBE

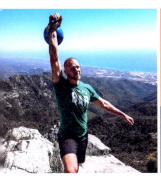
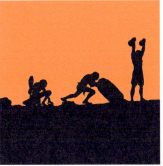
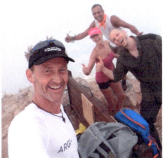

Add me: Facebook.com/taco.fleur or Facebook.com/coach.taco.fleur

Facebook.com/Cavemantraining or Facebook.com/Cavemantraining.Magazine
for up-to-date articles and news.

Please note that this material may not be reproduced or publicized elsewhere without the written consent of the author me@tacofleur.com.

If you bought this as a PDF/electronic copy, note that it is digitally signed and password protected with identifiable information.

All *Cavemantraining* owned images are copyrighted © *Cavemantraining*

Vouchers codes for discounts on the mobile app and *Udemy* course can be found toward the end of this book.

How to submit your assessment

You can submit your tasks or form check videos for free in any of our groups, usually I will respond myself, but there are plenty of other people who can also respond and help you with correct form and technique. Make sure you post "Kettlebell Guide for Beginners on Amazon by #cavemantraining" that way I know where what it belongs to and I will more put in more effort to reply to you myself. Following are the channels in which you can submit your video for assessment or ask questions:

- Kettlebell training for complete beginners (small group)
  www.facebook.com/groups/kettebells.for.beginners/
- Kettlebell training (large group)
  www.facebook.com/groups/KettlebellTraining/
- Kettlebell training (Reddit)
  www.reddit.com/r/kettlebell_training
- CrossFit WOD and Programming (aimed at crossfitters)
  www.facebook.com/groups/crossfit.wod.and.programming/
- Instagram (follow and tag me @realcavemantraining)
  www.instagram.com/realcavemantraining/

Without further ado, let's dive straight into the 21 days.

Day 1 Warming up and priming for kettlebell training

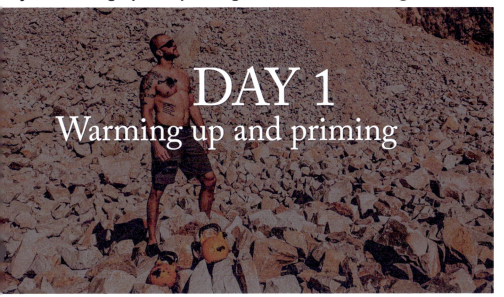

On day 1 you will learn how to warm up for kettlebell training and how super important it is to stay injury free. You will learn that mind-muscle connection is important for an effective and safe workout and that muscle priming is focussing on getting the muscles ready and assists in connecting with them.

I will take you through a **full-body warm up** and **muscle priming routine** for the kettlebell swing.

Dot points:

- Warming up for kettlebell training is super important
- Warm up to stay injury free
- Not one warm-up works for every workout or person
- Full-body warm-ups are best
- Mind-muscle connection is important for an effective and safe workout
- Muscle priming is focussing on getting the muscles ready and assists in connecting with them

Warming up for kettlebells

The full-body warm-up:

1. 10 x single leg hip circles one side
2. 10 x single leg hip circles other side
3. 10 x hip circles one way
4. 10 x hip circles other way

5. 10 x thoracic rotation one side
6. 10 x thoracic rotation other side
7. 10 x arm circled forward
8. 10 x arm circled backward
9. 10 to 20 x jumping jacks use high knees on the second round or complete after the jumping jacks

Single leg hip circles

To perform:

- Stand in a neutral stance
- Decide which hip to circle
- The leg of the non-circling hip should be locked (supporting leg)
- Firmly plant the foot on the ground
- Shift your weight onto the supporting leg
- Contract the gluteals on the supporting side to prevent the hip from dropping
- Lift the knee of the working leg through hip extension into starting position
- Pull the knee as high as possible
- Move the knee laterally out to the side and down creating a quarter of a circle
- Move the knee as for out to the side as possible and feel the stretch in the adductors
- If at this stage you struggle with balance then place the tippy toes on the ground for short support and continue the movement
- If you did not need support then finish the circle through extension and adduction which brings the leg straight under you but not touching the ground
- From there work on the next quarter circle by pulling the knee to the side of the supporting leg (adduction) and raising the knee (hip flexion)
- Feel the adductors working
- Make sure the hips don't drop or shift in any other direction while circling
- Finish the full circle with the last quarter and bring the knee up and back in front of you

Hip circles

To perform:

1. Stand in a neutral stance
2. Keep the spine straight throughout the movements
3. Keep the shoulders at the same level throughout the movement

4. Push the hips forward through hip hyperextension
5. Shift the hips to one side
6. Create slight hip flexion
7. Shift the hips to other side
8. And move the hips back into hip hyperextension
9. Repeat or circle back the other way

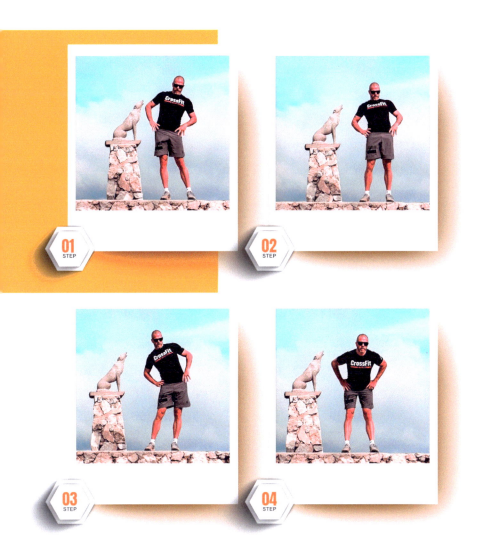

Thoracic rotation

Start with slow controlled movement
Pivot to protect the knees

To perform:

- Stand in a neutral stance
- Lockout the knees with the quads
- Lockout the hips with gluteals
- Think about one of your shoulders and the opposite buttock
  If you start with moving your left shoulder back then you would think about that and the right buttock
- Pull your shoulder back and down toward the buttock
- The movement starts from top vertebrae going down
- Pull the opposite shoulder toward the shoulder that is moving back
- Follow with the head in the direction you're moving
- Reach maximum safe range
- In a controlled movement come back into a neutral starting position
- Perform the same for the opposite side

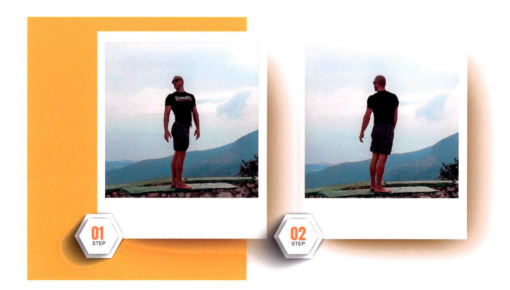

Arm circles

To perform:

- Stand in a neutral stance

- Let the arms hang beside the body
- Arms straight or slightly bend if shoulder flexibility is lacking
- Bring the arms back
- Follow through and create a circular motion forward with both arms

You can also go the opposite direction.

Jumping jacks

Go easy on the overhead position and ease into it as you get warmer.

To perform:

- Stand in a neutral stance
- Let the arms hang beside the body
- Bring the feet apart
- At the same time bring the arms up
- Bring the feet back in
- At the same time bring the arms back beside the body-part
- Repeat

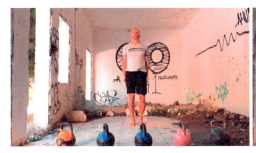
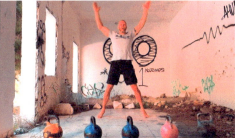

Duration

Your whole warm-up should take 5 to 6 minutes but that also depends on the weather, your state, etc. Increase duration as required.

Task

Your first task is to complete the warm-up as described above, you can do just one round or do more.

Submission

You can film your warm-up for feedback. Submit your video in any way possible. See chapter on *How to submit your assessment*.

Mind-muscle connection and muscle priming

MMC is all about connecting with the right muscles to perform the movement or stabilize for the movement, it is also used to relax the muscles that could be doing part of the work (isolation). Muscle priming is getting the muscles ready that will be doing the work and assists with MMC.

Muscle priming routine for the kettlebell swing:

- Prone bent single leg raises
- Kneeling hip extensions
- Prone back hyperextensions
- Quarter squats
- Calf raises
- Lat pull down
- Scapulae adduction

You're working out to put your muscles under stress. The more muscles you incorporate in your exercise the bigger results you're going to get. Recruit more muscles with MMC.

Prone bent single leg raises

Prone is lying face down.

You're connecting with your gluteus maximus.

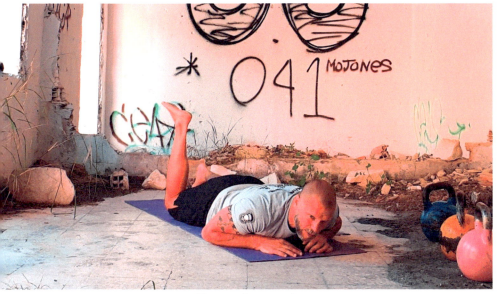
Knee on the ground

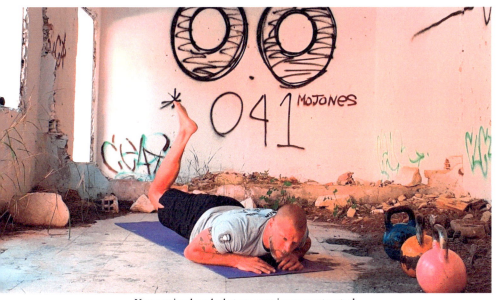
Knee raised and gluteus maximus contracted

Kneeling hip extensions

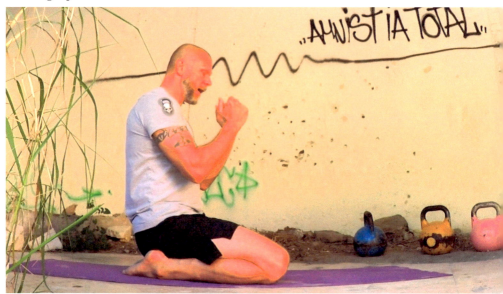
Kneeling position

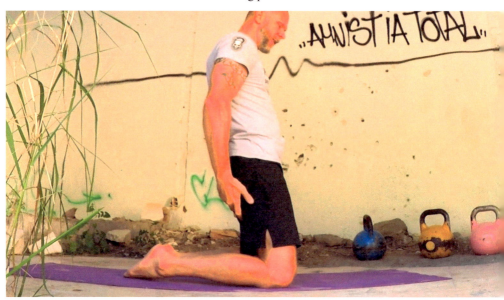
Hip extension with focus on the hamstrings

Prone back hyperextensions

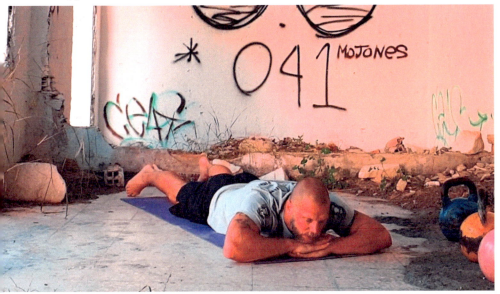

Laying prone

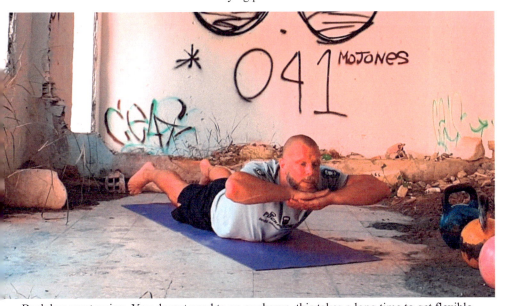

Back hyperextension. You do not need to go as shown, this takes a long time to get flexible. The objective is to connect with the back muscles which stay rigid to protect the spine during the swing.

Quarter squats

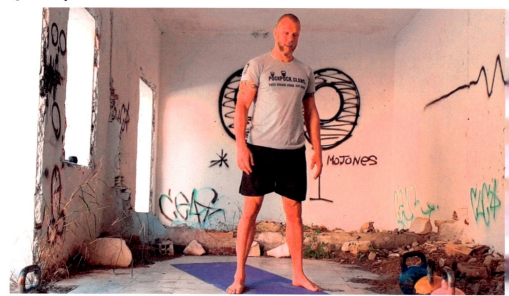
Starting position

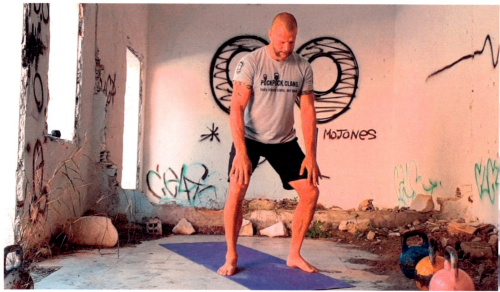
Quarter squat to connect with the area which will extend the knees and move the hips forward.

Calf raises

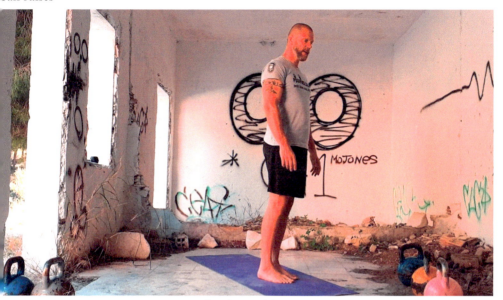

Starting position

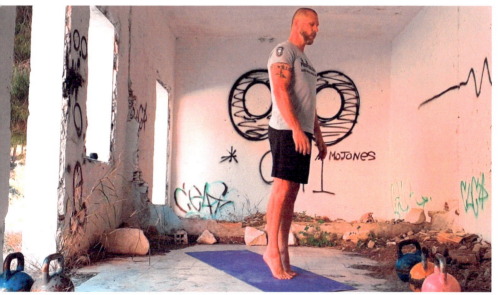

Calf raise to connect with the area which will work to keep the knees above the ankles during the swing.

Lat pull down

Hold on to something and lean to the side, then contract the lat and pull the elbow into the ribs.

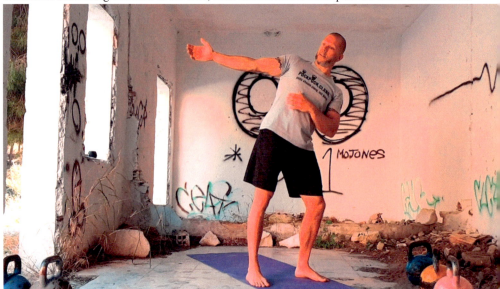

Lean to the side while holding on

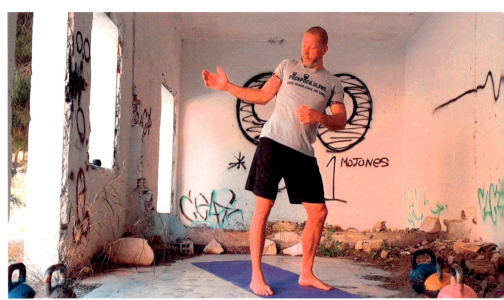

Pull the elbow in to the side and connect with the lats to connect with the area that will be pulling down to protect the shoulders during the swing with slight contraction.

Scapulae adduction

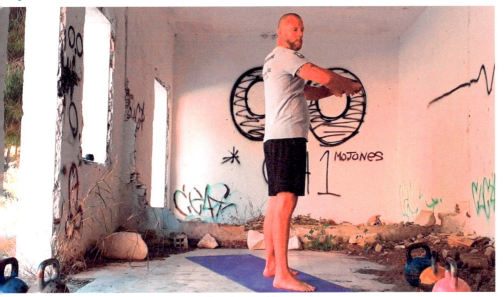

Starting position

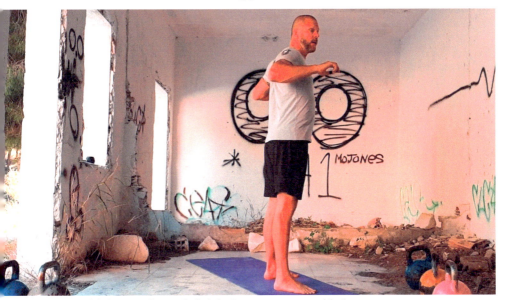

Pull the shoulder blades together and slightly down to connect with the area you want to contract at the top of the swing and slightly during.

Task

Your second task is to complete the muscle priming as per below.

- 5 x prone bent single leg raises each side
- 10 x kneeling hip extension
- 5 x prone back hyperextensions
- 10 seconds static back hyperextension
- 10 x quarter squats
- 10 x calf raises
- 5 x lat pull down each side
- 10 x scapulae adduction

Repeat twice.

Submission

You can film your priming for feedback. Submit your video in any way possible. See chapter on *How to submit your assessment*.

Day 2 Stretching and mobility for kettlebell training

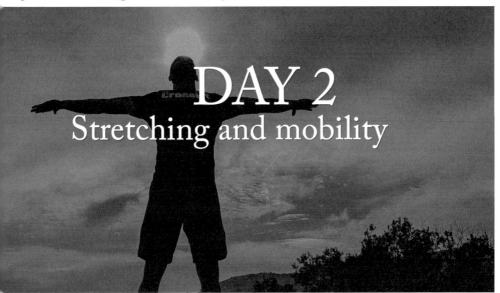

On day 2 you will learn how to stretch and perform some mobility work to increase performance and reduce chance of injury.

Stretching and mobility work is generally performed after working out, however, I recommend you incorporate it as much as you can, before, during, and after.

Dot points:

- Pulse into positions when you're still warming up
- Keep your stretches dynamic at the start of your session
- Increase time in the stretch as you progress through your session
- Internally rotate while kneeling to protect the knee
- Progress step-by-step into the Jefferson curl over a long period of time
- You do not want to feel stress in your lumbar
- The goal of an exercise can change by how you program and perform it
- You never want to feel any torque on the knees

Movements/stretches:

- Reverse lunge
- Reverse lunge arms overhead
- Reverse lunge and twist

- Runners lunge and twist
- Kneeling
- Kneeling and hip extension
- Kneeling and hip flexion with arms overhead
- Kneeling with hip abduction
- Jefferson curl
- Pigeon

Reverse lunge

To perform:

- Stand in a neutral stance
- Decide which leg is going to be supporting and which one is going to lunge back
- Shift your weight onto the supporting side
- Lunge back through sliding or hovering the foot back in position
- The distance back is as far back as possible while keeping the knee above or slightly behind the ankle at the front
- Keep the weight at the front as much as possible
- Use the back leg for balance only
- Aim to gently touch the ground with the back knee
- Spend a short moment in the full lunge position and press the ball of the lunging foot into the ground
- Gently push the hips forward to benefit from the hip flexor stretch
- Your weight is still on the supporting leg
- Press the supporting foot into the ground and contract the quads and gluteals to come back up

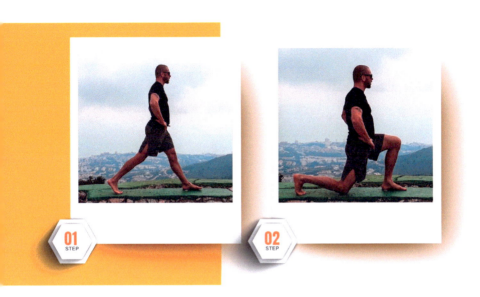

Reverse lunge arms overhead

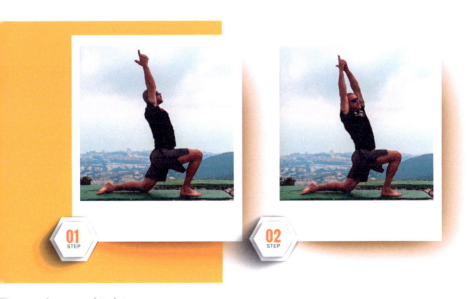

Reverse lunge and twist

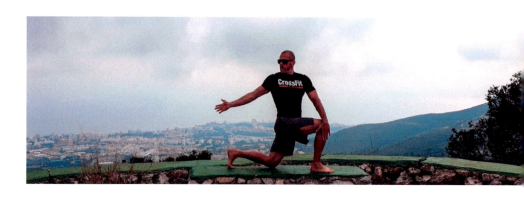

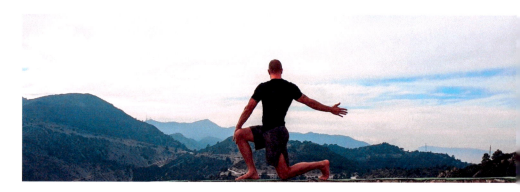

Benefits:

- Strength
- Stability
- Hip flexor stretch
- Ball of the foot stretch

Runners lunge and twist

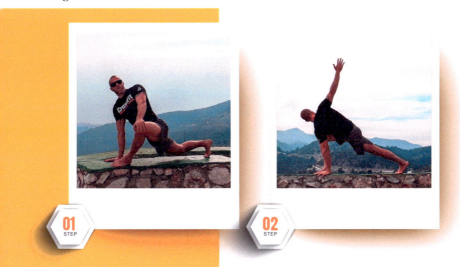

01 STEP

02 STEP

Kneeling

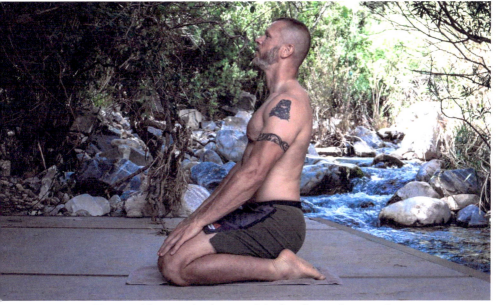

Your goal is to get the dorsum of the feet flat on the ground.

Kneeling and hip extension

You're working up to kneeling and leaning back with hip extension to get a deeper hip flexor stretch.

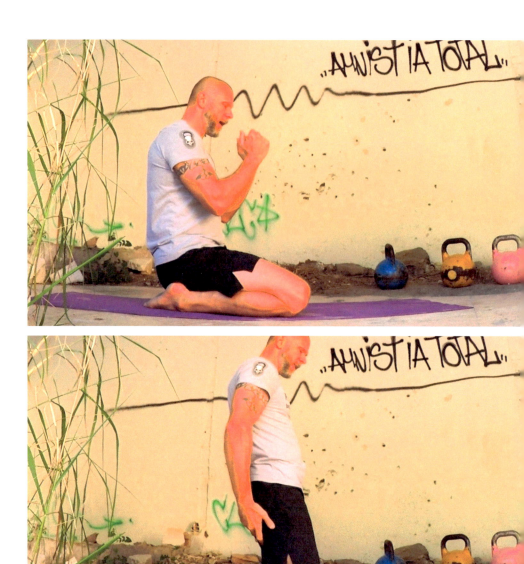

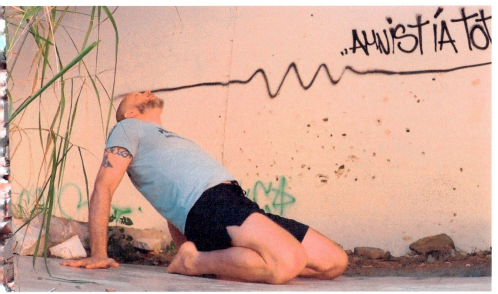

This is where you want to work up to or if you already have the flexibility go straight into this pose.

Kneeling and hip flexion with arms overhead

Same as above staring kneeling position but with the arms overhead, if possible, with the palms together.

Kneeling with hip abduction

Same as above starting kneeling position but with the knees further apart.

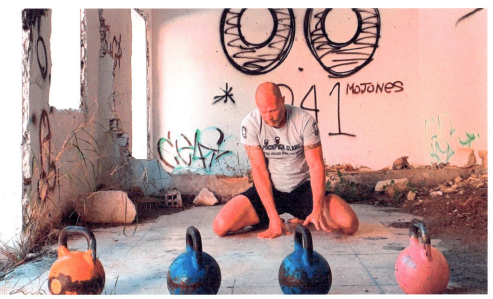

This position is to get into the hip adductors.

Jefferson curl

Step-by-step

- Neutral stance
- Let your arms relax and hang
- Gently press the heels into the ground creating slight tension between the ankles and hips
- Slightly contract the glutes to keep the pelvis aligned vertically
- Start flexing/curling at the top between the thoracic and cervical (neck) spine
- All movement in the spine will be from the top down vertebra by vertebra
- Let your shoulders droop forward
- Your head comes along through flexion at the cervical
- Connect with the muscles at the back and feel each vertebra enter near max flexion
- Continue moving down the thoracic spine
- Leave the lumbar alone and without flexion
- Move to the hips and create hip flexion
- Actively pull the pelvis down toward the ground
- Continue to near max range of hip flexion
- Don't go to the point of pain in the hamstrings
- Keep the legs vertically aligned
- Reach for your toes with the hands
- Don't rush the range
- Time to come back up
- Reverse everything you've done
- Start at the hips
- Pull the pelvis up from the bottom with the hamstrings and adductor magnus
- Pull the pelvis up from the top with the gluteus maximus
- Follow through with each vertebra until in neutral vertical stance

Feel the muscles, engage the muscles, connect with the muscles.

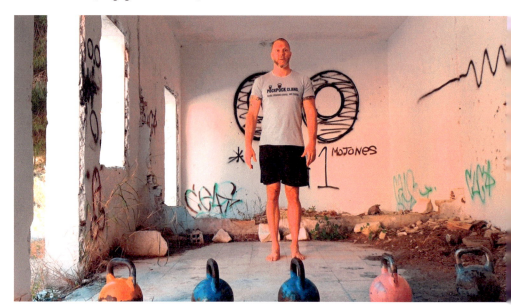

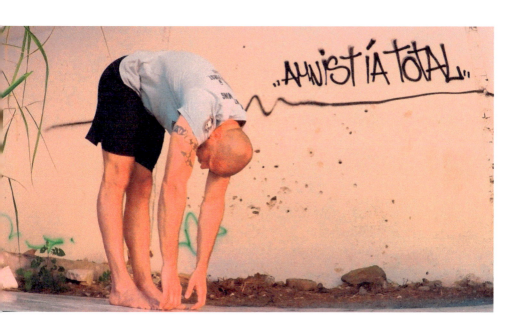

Pigeon

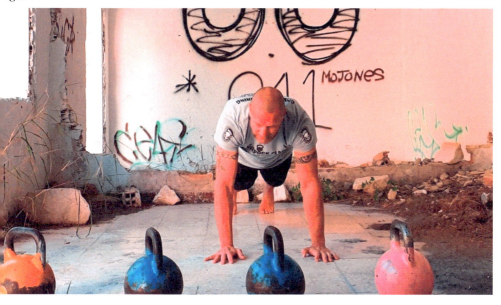

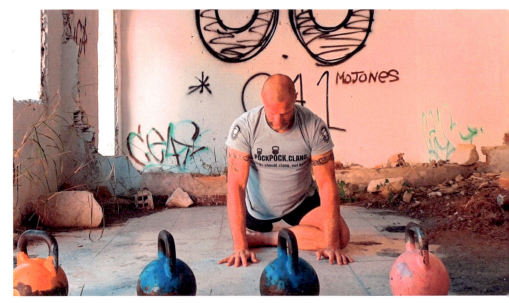

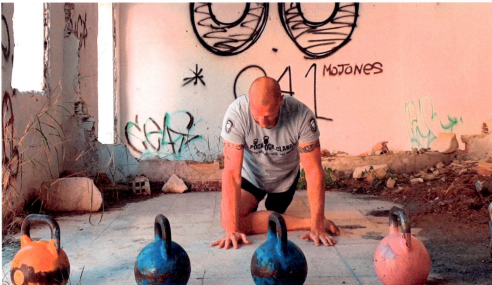

Great stretch to get into the glutes but avoid torque on the knee and create external hip rotation to protect the knees.

Mobility
Mobility is a combination of flexibility, strength, stability, coordination, proprioception, and more, in short, it's defined by how easily you can perform the movement and what ROM can you reach. Slow down your movements to focus on mobility.

Feet
Your feet are super important for balance, performance, stability, spend time on your feet. It's

recommended not to train with kettlebells in runners. Ankle circles, calf raises, and Hindu squats are great to train and work on the feet.

Task

Your third task is to complete some stretching and mobility work as per below.

Warm up first

First round:

- 2 x reverse lunge both sides
- 4 x alternating pigeon
- 5 x reverse lunge arms overhead both sides
- 3 x Jefferson curl
- 5 x reverse lunge and twist both sides
- 4 x alternating pigeon
- 3 x runners lunge and twist both sides
- 5 x kneeling and hip extension
- 5 x kneeling and hip flexion with arms overhead
- 3 x Jefferson curl

The first round was more dynamic, moving in and out of positions, and your second round will be slightly longer holds at the end of movements. All movements are to be performed slowly and controlled.

Second round:

- 2 x reverse lunge both sides
- 3 x alternating pigeon
- 2 x reverse lunge arms overhead both sides
- 2 x Jefferson curl
- 2 x reverse lunge and twist both sides
- 3 x alternating pigeon
- 2 x runners lunge and twist both sides
- 4 x kneeling and hip extension
- 3 x kneeling and hip flexion with arms overhead
- 2 x Jefferson curl

Third round:

- Reverse lunge both sides
- Pigeon both sides
- Reverse lunge arms overhead both sides

- Jefferson curl
- Reverse lunge and twist both sides
- Alternating pigeon
- Runners lunge and twist both sides
- Kneeling and hip flexion with arms overhead
- Jefferson curl

10 to 15-second hold for each position.

Submission

You can film your stretching and mobility work for feedback. Submit your video in any way possible. See chapter on How to submit your assessment.

Day 3 Kettlebell anatomy and grip

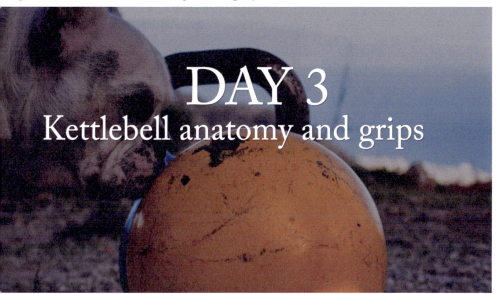

On **day 3 you will learn** about the anatomy of the kettlebell and grips which is the first important information you should know to progress with your kettlebell training. I'll also cover some exercises for wrist strength.

There are over 25 kettlebell grips, I will cover the common kettlebell grips:

- Hook grip
- Closed hook grip
- Double hand grip
- Closed double hand grip

Kettlebell anatomy:

- Handle
- Horn(s)
- Window
- Bell
- Base

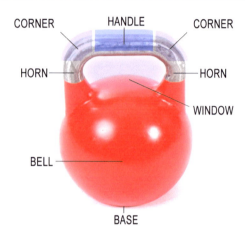

ILLUSTRATED: COMPETITION KETTLEBELL

Grip is usually the first point of failure on high reps snatches or swings with correct technique.

Other points:

- A kettlebell grip should be loose but tight enough to hold on to the kettlebell
- You can work your grip strength by holding the kettlebell in the tips of the fingers
- Wrist strength is often overlooked in training
- You can work on lateral wrist flexion with the kettlebell on the ground and base pointing up
- When you first start training make sure you ease into reps and weight
- Progress slowly and rest enough so you can keep training
- You can work wrist flexion and extension while standing and letting the bell hang next to you
- Stretch your forearms after working out
- Grip is relaxed at the top of the swing

You can download a FREE PDF with over 25 kettlebell grips in it from our website here.

Day 4 Safely lifting the kettlebell with a squat

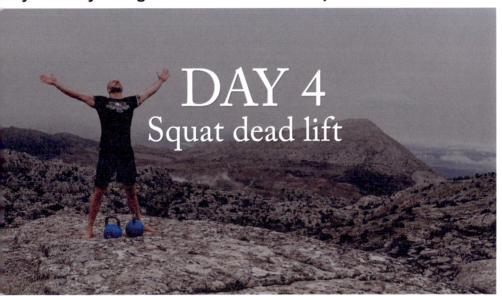

Dot points:

- Deadlift means that the weight starts dead on the ground and is then lifted
- Dead means that the weight is not moving
- Shoulders high and hips low with the squat while pushing the hips toward the ground
- Maintain good aligned between the three joints during the squat
- The knee is a hinge joint that only flexes and extends
- Don't reach out for the weight
- Protect the spine during lifts with a rigid structure
- Perform the hang lift to work on flexibility and range
- If the shoulders come low while the hips stay high then you are not squatting but hip hinging
- Range and technique before weight and reps

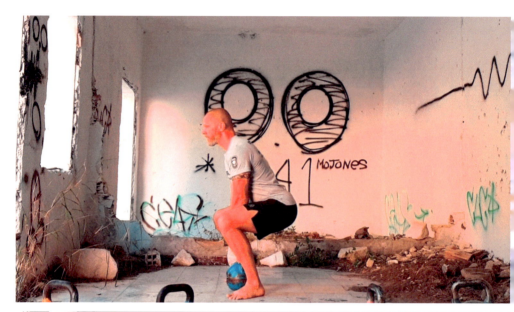
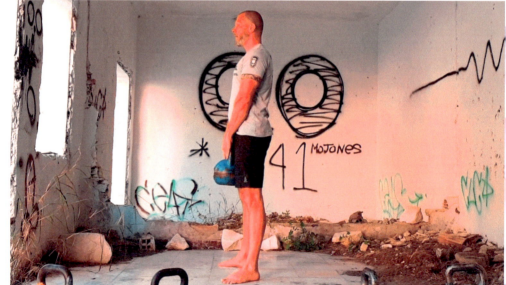

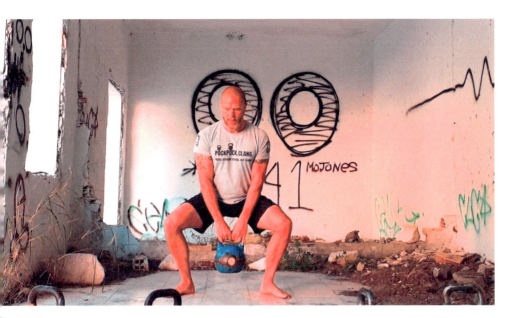

Task

Your fourth task is to complete several sets of the squat dead lift as per below.

Warm up first.

If your form and technique is already close to good then perform 8 reps of the dead lift otherwise regress to 4 reps of the hang lift.

Perform the reps on one side and then rest for 15 to 30 seconds or do 1 minute of mobility work like for example some dynamic pigeon, kneeling hip extensions (focus on working butt to the ground), or reverse lunge and pulse with arms overhead. After the rest you perform a set on the other side. Perform 8 to 12 sets in total.

If you've used your rest time for mobility work then you've already done your stretching for the day, otherwise, end with some stretching.

Submission

You can film your squat dead lift for feedback. Submit your video in any way possible. See chapter on How to submit your assessment.

Day 5 Safely lifting the kettlebell with a hip hinge

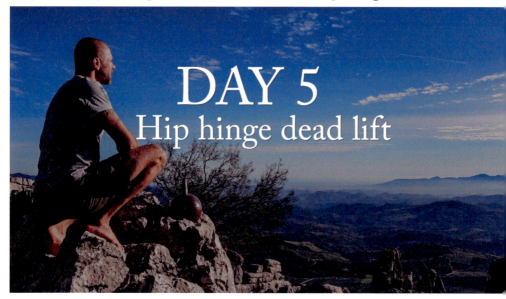

Dot points:

- The hip hinge is the most common movement used for deadlifting
- The hip hinge is performed with one or two joints
- The knees stay above the ankles when hinging
- The top of the pelvis is pulled up with the gluteus maximus
- The pull at the bottom of the pelvis is created by the hamstrings (3 muscles) and the adductor magnus
- First master the bodyweight hip hinge before adding weight to the movement
- The weight should be positioned under the shoulder while in the hinge
- Do not bend the back to reach for the weight
- Perform the hip hinge hang lift if you're working on range (3HL)
- Don't hold your breath during the lift
- Brace your core to protect the spine
- Keep your spine straight throughout the lift
- The hip hinge deadlift is better to be performed for strength with slow focussed movement

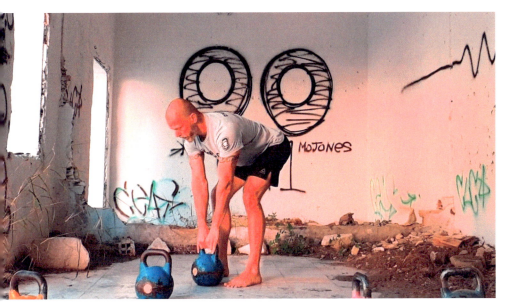

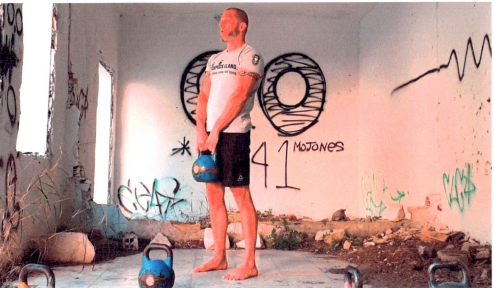

Task

Your fifth task is to complete several sets of the hip hinge dead lift as per below.

Warm up first.

If your form and technique is already close to good then perform 8 reps of the dead lift otherwise regress to 4 reps of the hang lift.

Perform the reps on one side and then rest for 15 to 30 seconds or do 1 minute of mobility work like for example some dynamic pigeon, kneeling hip extensions (focus on working butt to the ground), or reverse lunge and pulse with arms overhead. After the rest you perform a set on the other side. Perform 8 to 12 sets in total.

If you've used your rest time for mobility work then you've already done your stretching for the day, otherwise end with some stretching.

Submission
You can film your hip hinge dead lift for feedback. Submit your video in any way possible. See chapter on How to submit your assessment.

Day 6 Assisted kettlebell clean

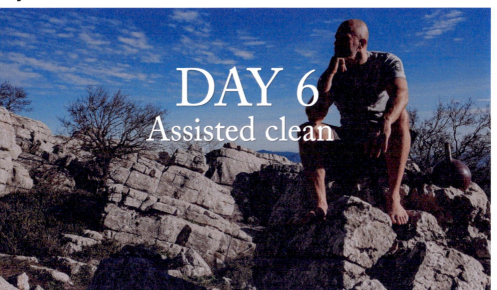

Dot points:

- The assisted clean is performed with a squat
- This drill is super important and will flow through in more advanced progressions
- A clean brings a weight from lower into racking position
- The assisted clean is to be performed slow and controlled to learn the movement and positions
- Eventually you will progress to an explosive movement
- Cleans are explosive apart from the assisted clean which is a drill
- The assisted clean is to teach hand insertion and racking
- Raise the weight with a box if you're working on flexibility
- Open the hand and let the bell come around the hand
- Skip the palm to avoid friction
- No need to look at the weight you know where it is
- Elbow pulled in tight on the rack
- A broken wrist grip is where the line is broken at the wrist
- Racking and bell pressure on the forearm requires some conditioning
- Don't overtrain but gradually increase duration and reps
- Don't put the non working arm/hand on the body during a lift
- Create good form and technique
- Create good habits
- Drill the insert on the ground
- Take note of where the arm should be positioned after the insert
- Use a weight easy enough to handle (light to medium)

- Progress slowly step by step
- Drill drill drill

Assisted clean:
- Squat
- Hook grip
- Lift
- Full extension
- Slight curl
- Assist with the other hand
- Lift the weight up
- Open the hand
- Roll the kettlebell over
- Hand insert
- Rack
- Reverse with assistance
- Pull out
- Hook grip
- Full arm extension into squat
- Lower the weight to dead

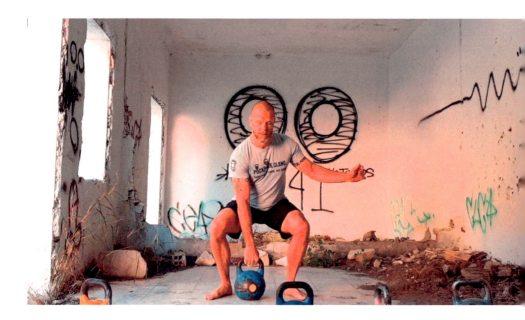

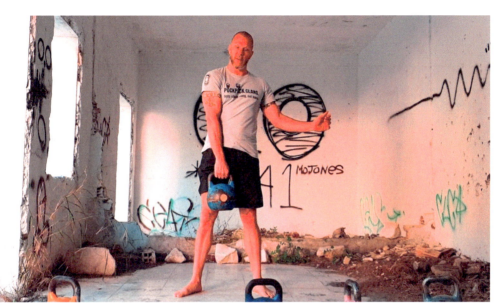
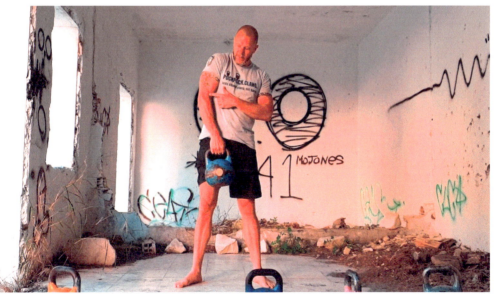

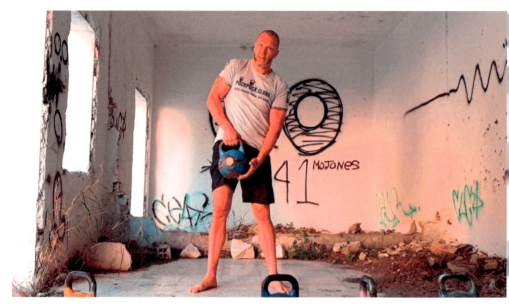
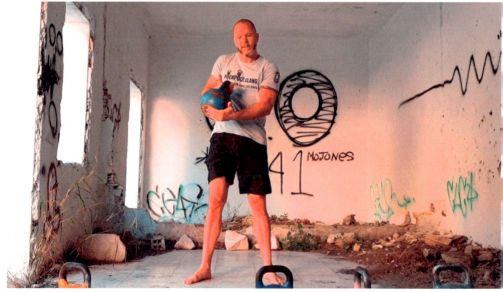

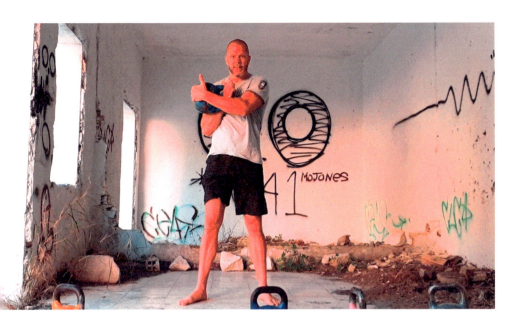

Double hand dead swing clean

The double hand clean is great for beginners but also used with heavy weights or in kettlebell sport where endurance and energy preservation is important. You should wait till hip hinge swing is covered before attempting this one.

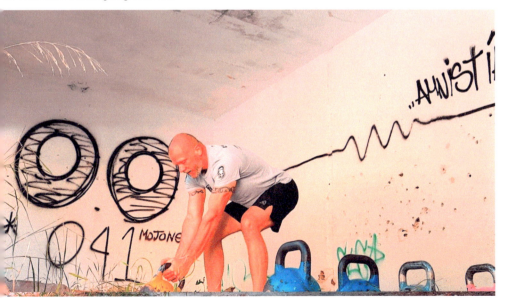

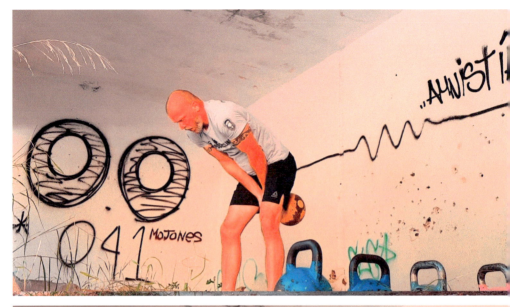

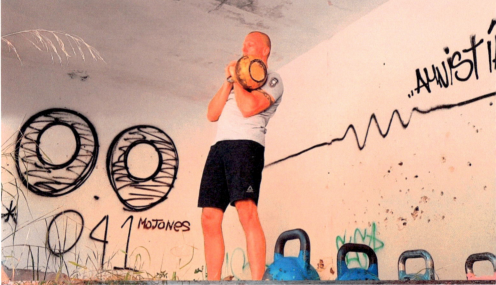

Task

Your sixth task is to complete several sets of the assisted clean as per below.

If in the previous chapters you were doing hang lifts then also perform hang lifts here instead of the dead lift.

Perform four slow reps on one side and repeat on the other. Each rep should take about 10 to 15 seconds. Rest if required, then repeat, work for 4 to 6 minutes. Repeat this drill for as long as you need to master and understand the movement. You can do this 3 times a day with plenty of space in

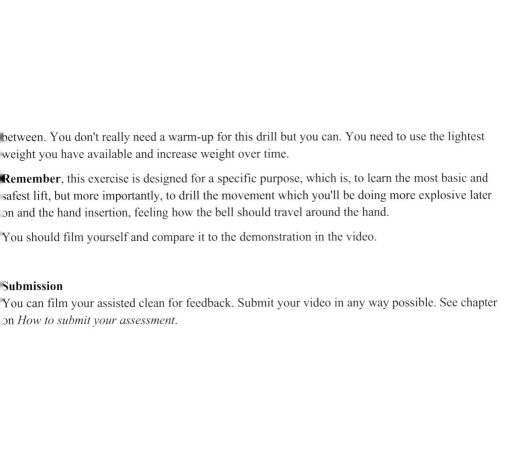

between. You don't really need a warm-up for this drill but you can. You need to use the lightest weight you have available and increase weight over time.

Remember, this exercise is designed for a specific purpose, which is, to learn the most basic and safest lift, but more importantly, to drill the movement which you'll be doing more explosive later on and the hand insertion, feeling how the bell should travel around the hand.

You should film yourself and compare it to the demonstration in the video.

Submission

You can film your assisted clean for feedback. Submit your video in any way possible. See chapter on *How to submit your assessment*.

Day 7 Kettlebell squat swing

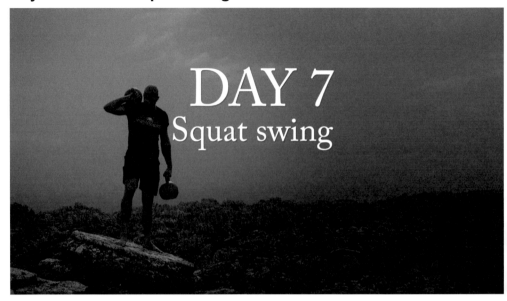

Dot points:

- The kettlebell swing is one of the most popular kettlebell exercises
- There is so much more to kettlebell training than just the swing
- There are many different types of kettlebell swings
- The squat swing is controversial
- A swing is good if its safe and works towards your goals
- It is important to know why you're doing an exercise
- You should also learn the hip hinge swing
- Understand the differences between squat and hip hinge
- The squat swing uses more of the anterior muscles and is less stress on the lower back
- The hip hinge is more isolation of the gluteus maximus and provides more stress on the back (not always a bad thing)
- In the swing your arms are just a pendulum with your shoulder being the pivot
- The only swing that is a shoulder raise is the *American swing*
- Shoulders should be slightly pulled back and down
- Don't pull the kettlebell up with the shoulders
- Drive the weight up with the power from your legs
- To start you bump the weight out and don't worry how high it comes
- If the kettlebell comes too high then the weight is probably too light
- The weight is too heavy if it does not come higher than the hips
- The kettlebell should be a direct extension of your arms at all times
- There should be no bobbing at the end or top of the swing
- If you can see the ground at the bottom of your swing you're probably hip hinging

- You can also start your swing with a dead start (dead swing)
- You need more flexibility for the dead start
- Don't over reach for the kettlebell
- Whether you keep your arms straight or bent depends on the trajectory of the kettlebell
- If the kettlebell trajectory is away from you then the arms should remain straight
- If the kettlebell trajectory is up then you can bent your arms
- Guiding the kettlebell away from you adds more back muscle recruitment
- Bent arm with the trajectory being out and away creates tension/tugs on the elbow flexors

Kettlebell squat swing:

1. Bump the weight out to start
2. Let the weight freely drop down
3. Guide the weight between the legs and towards the ground
4. Bend the three joints for the squat
5. Keep the shoulders high
6. Look ahead
7. Pull the weight back up
8. Come back upright
9. Push the heels into the ground
10. Pull the knees back
11. Extend the hips
12. Let the weight come up and forward
13. Come into full extension
14. The weight reach about chest height
15. Let the weight drop back down
16. Repeat

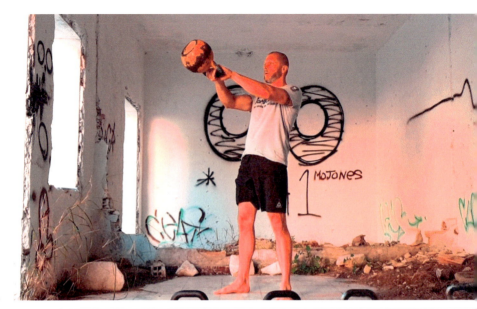

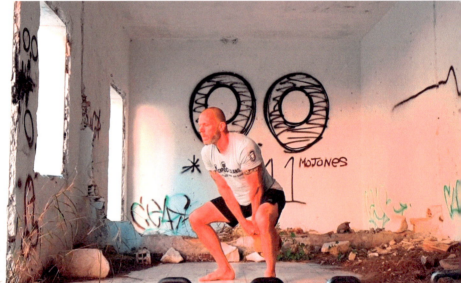

Task

Your seventh task is to complete several sets of the squat swing with double arm as per below.

Start with a dead start if you have the flexibility, if you don't, remember to work on your flexibility.

Pick a weight that allows you to easily get the kettlebell till about chest height but not higher. Pick a weight that requires you to activate the glutes and hammies (hip extensors) but not fatigue them,

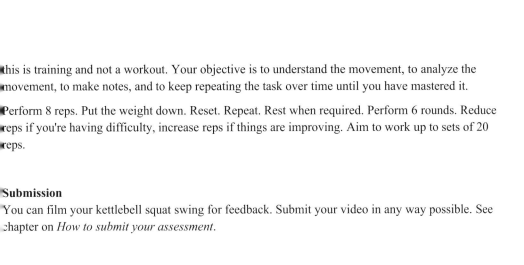

this is training and not a workout. Your objective is to understand the movement, to analyze the movement, to make notes, and to keep repeating the task over time until you have mastered it.

Perform 8 reps. Put the weight down. Reset. Repeat. Rest when required. Perform 6 rounds. Reduce reps if you're having difficulty, increase reps if things are improving. Aim to work up to sets of 20 reps.

Submission

You can film your kettlebell squat swing for feedback. Submit your video in any way possible. See chapter on *How to submit your assessment*.

Day 8 Kettlebell hip hinge swing

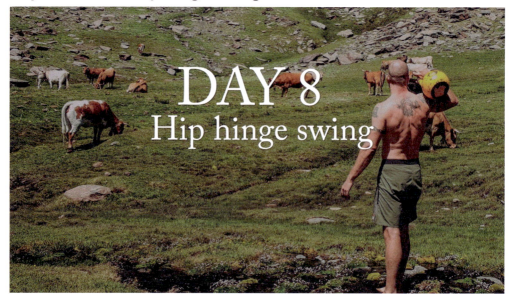

On day 8 you will learn the most common version of the kettlebell swing and I'll talk about how to avoid back aches, what muscles to active and why, and many more tips that are commonly overlooked and will result in back aches when not implemented.

I will also demonstrate how to start the kettlebell swing safety several different ways.

Dot points:
- The hip hinge swing is the most common kettlebell swing
- The movement is wrong when the hip hinge swing is performed with a squat
- Hip hinge and insert
- Pull out and direct the weight forward
- Look ahead at the top of the swing
- Look at the ground in-front at the bottom of the swing
- The hip hinge swing involves two joints for power
- Hips and knees
- The swing can be performed with one joint
- With the hips only it is called the stiff-legged swing
- The swing is going to hurt your back if you do not engage the right muscles intended for the movement
- The right muscles are; gluteus maximus; hamstrings; adductor magnus

- Work on MMC if you experience lower back pain
- Look at technique
- Review programming (reps/weight/rest)
- To protect the lower back you should not follow the kettlebell
- Direct the weight to the back
- Don't let the weight abruptly be stopped by your groin
- Don't let the kettlebell hit your tailbone
- Film and analyze yourself
- Film and ask for form check
- The swing can be started with a dead start (dead swing)
- Do low reps when just starting out
- Stop when you have pain and review muscle priming/MMC
- Focus on technique
- You can breathe twice during the swing
- Breathe out at the top and end
- You can breathe once during the swing
- Breathe in on the way down
- Breathe out on the way up
- Don't hold your breath

Kettlebell hip hinge swing:

1. Squat dead lift
2. Bump it out
3. Delay the hinge till the weight is at the right position
4. Insert
5. The weight should come through about knee height
6. Direct the weight to the back
7. Prevent bobbing of the kettlebell
8. Pull the weight back out with the muscles intended
9. Direct the weight forward
10. Come into full extension

11. Wait for the weight to drop back down
12. Delay hip flexion
13. Insert
14. Repeat

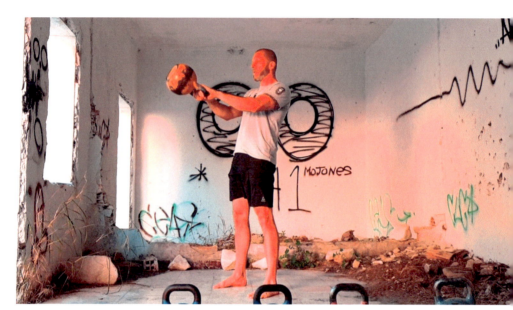

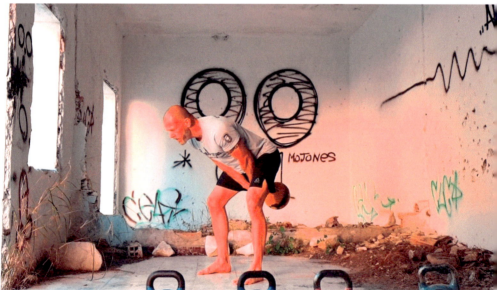

Compare the hip hinge to the squat

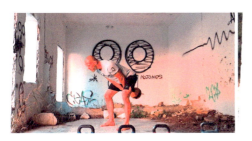 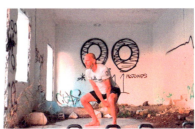

Task

Your eighth task is to complete several sets of the hip hinge swing with double arm as per below.

Start with a dead start if you have the flexibility, if you don't, remember to work on your flexibility.

Pick a weight that allows you to easily get the kettlebell till about chest height but not higher. Pick a weight that requires you to activate the glutes and hammies (hip extensors) but not fatigue them, this is training and not a workout. Your objective is to understand the movement, to analyze the movement, to make notes, and to keep repeating the task over time until you have mastered it.

Perform 6 reps. Put the weight down. Reset. Repeat. Rest when required. Perform 8 rounds. Reduce reps if you're having difficulty, increase reps if things are improving. Aim to work up to sets of 20 reps.

Submission

You can film your hip hinge swing for feedback. Submit your video in any way possible. See chapter on How to submit your assessment.

Day 9 Kettlebell pendulum swing

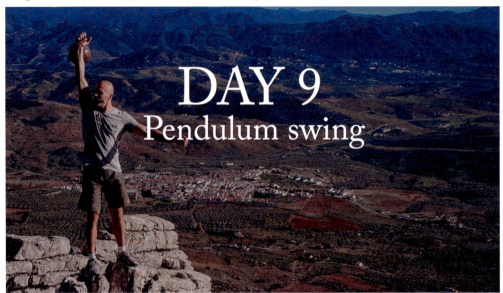

On day 9 you will learn a version of the kettlebell swing that is more advanced but once mastered will open up a whole new world of kettlebell training to you. This version of the swing provides the least resistance to the body and is great for high volume swings. This swing also can improve your clean a lot and gets you ready for snatches in the future.

Dot points:
- There are 3 main movements to perform the swing
- Squat; Hip hinge; Pendulum
- The pendulum swing comes from kettlebell sport
- The pendulum swing is usually performed with one arm
- Make space for the bell
- Stay connected
- Go with the flow
- Don't resist the weight
- This is a push whereas the other two movements are a pull
- Push the arms forward
- Great swing for high volume reps
- Each swing has their own reason for doing them
- The pendulum swing is great for the clean

- There are many different ways to perform the pendulum swing
- The pendulum swing provides the least amount of stress on the body
- Know when to use one over the other

Kettlebell pendulum swing:
- Bump the weight out
- The knees bent
- The arms connect with the body
- The hips are coming back to prevent an abrupt stop
- The knees extend to prevent an abrupt stop
- The shoulders are coming down (hip hinge) to prevent an abrupt stop
- The weight comes back through gravity
- Follow the bell with the hips
- Keep the arms connected
- Push with the hips
- Perform slight hip hyperextension if flexibility allows (stay connected longer)
- The weight does not need to come to any specific height
- Let the weight come back in and through
- Repeat

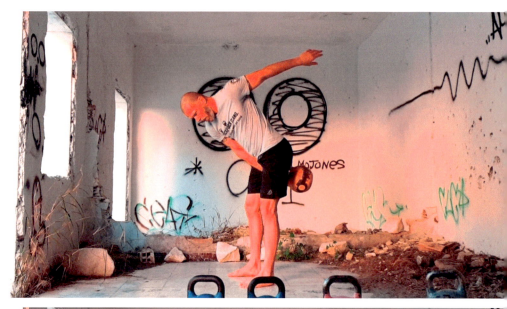
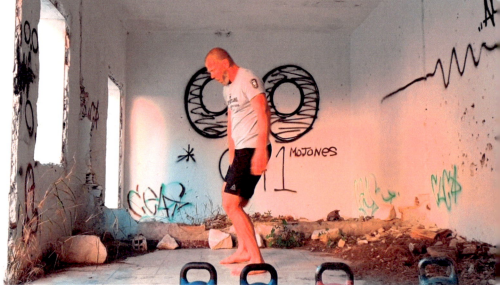

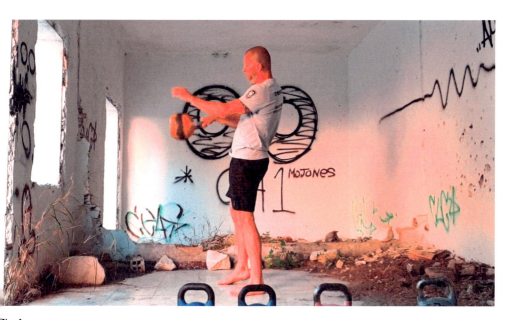

Task

Your ninth task is to complete several sets of the pendulum swing with double arm as per below, but if you find that the swing works better for you with single arm that is fine too, just split the number of reps in half for each side.

Start with a dead start if you have the flexibility, if you don't, remember to work on your flexibility.

Pick a weight that is close to 1/3 heavier than what you've been using for the hip hinge swings. Your objective is to understand the movement, to analyze the movement, to make notes, and to keep repeating the task over time until you have mastered it.

Perform 20 reps. Put the weight down. Reset. Repeat. Rest when required. Perform 6 rounds. Reduce reps if you're having difficulty, increase reps if things are improving. Aim to work up to one set of 60.

Submission

You can film your pendulum swing for feedback. Submit your video in any way possible. See chapter on How to submit your assessment.

Day 10 Double arm swing clean

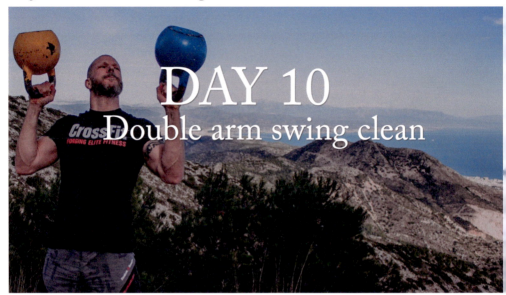

On day 10 you will learn the double arm swing clean which is great to transition into other movements like the squat, press, halo, etc. In other words, once you know this type of clean you can start stringing movements together and create flows.

I will introduce you to some concepts that will help prevent injury when you move on to more complex kettlebell cleans.

The double arm swing clean is great to transition into other movements like the squat, press, halo, etc. In other words, once you know this type of clean you can start stringing movements together and create flows.

Dot points:

- When people refer to a 'clean' they will refer to the most common clean 'they' taught you
- There are many different types of cleans
- Getting specific with naming avoids confusing as to what is asked of the athlete
- Start; Dead swing clean; Swing clean; Hang clean; Dead clean
- Movement; Squat; Hip hinge; Pendulum
- There are over 70 different types/variations of the kettlebell clean
- With a clean you want to keep the weight close to you
- You want the trajectory to be up
- Keeping the elbows in will keep the weight close
- Don't cast the weight out and away from you
- Let the weight drop

- Sometimes a heavier weight for the clean will force you to use correct technique

Double arm swing clean:

- Bump the weight out or start with the weight dead
- Perform the movement to drive the weight up
- Transition the hands from grip on the handle to grip around the bell
- Keep the thumbs pointing up within the window
- Base of the bell should be up but not completely horizontal
- Bring the weight to the chest
- Drop the weight
- Transition into double hand grip
- Move into the backswing
- Repeat

Beginners option is to keep the index finger and thumb closed on both sides which creates a ring around the handle that can be slid across to the horns. Doing so will prevent the need to let go of the kettlebell which can sometimes be daunting for beginners. The grip needs to be loose to be able to slide it across the handle and horns.

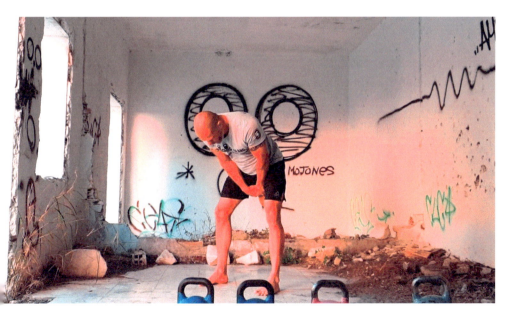

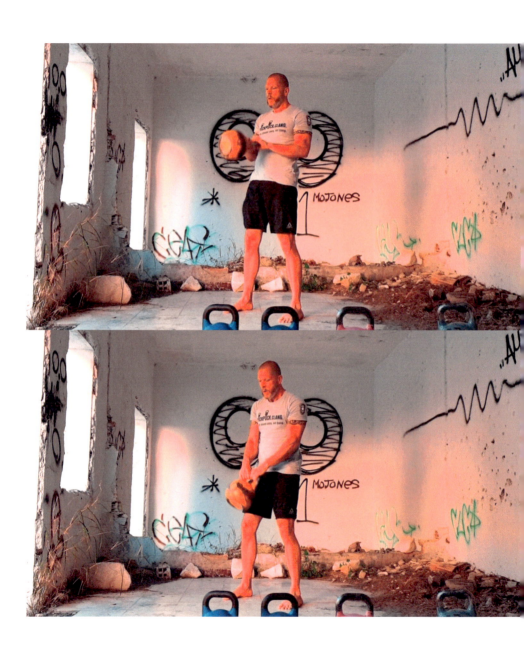

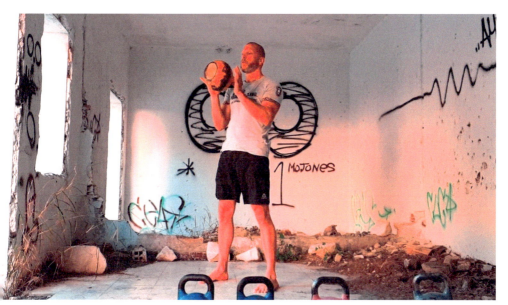

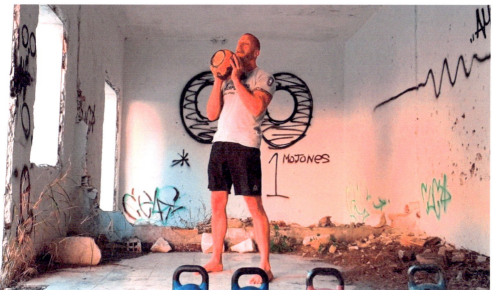

Safety

Catch the weight away from you. When starting out that distance should be great and decreasing as you become more comfortable. If you're not comfortable performing this clean you can just put the weight safely down and lift the bell from the ground in a squat position.

Task

Your tenth task is to complete several sets of the double arm swing clean as per below.

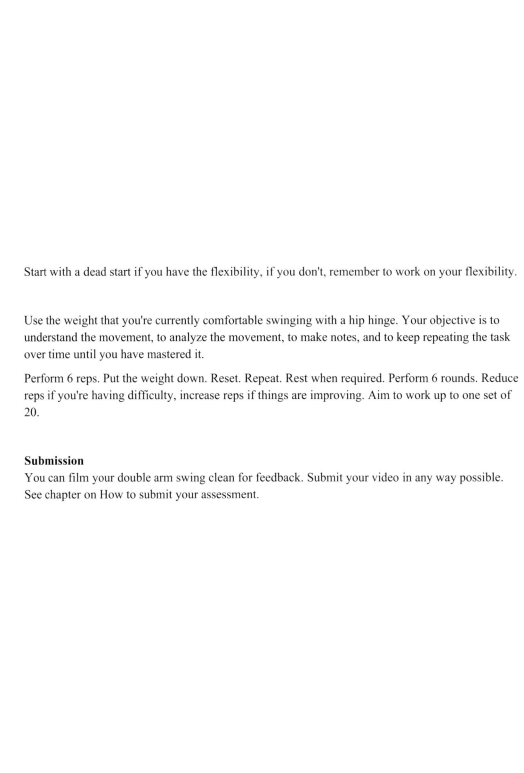

Start with a dead start if you have the flexibility, if you don't, remember to work on your flexibility.

Use the weight that you're currently comfortable swinging with a hip hinge. Your objective is to understand the movement, to analyze the movement, to make notes, and to keep repeating the task over time until you have mastered it.

Perform 6 reps. Put the weight down. Reset. Repeat. Rest when required. Perform 6 rounds. Reduce reps if you're having difficulty, increase reps if things are improving. Aim to work up to one set of 20.

Submission
You can film your double arm swing clean for feedback. Submit your video in any way possible. See chapter on How to submit your assessment.

Day 11 Kettlebell dead clean

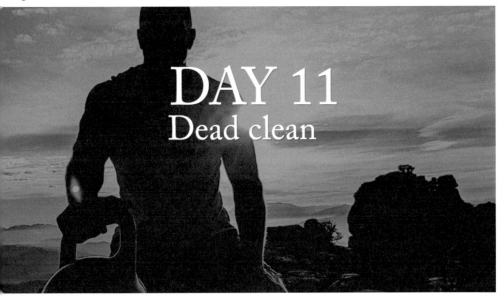

On day 11 you will learn the kettlebell dead clean which is a very explosive movement and great to add to your training. This version of the clean is very similar to the barbell clean in CrossFit. This is where it becomes obvious why you've been drilling the assisted clean.

I will demonstrate this movement step by step and talk about the muscles that need to be engaged and so much more.

Dot points:

- You'll need a heavier kettlebell for this exercise
- The clean brings a kettlebell from a lower position into racking position
- Perform the squat movement to perform this exercise
- This exercise is what you've been drilling the assisted clean for
- The bell comes around the hand and not over the fist
- Make sure you've been drilling the assisted clean
- If you're struggling with the dead clean then drill the assisted clean more
- The weight travel directly up in one straight line looking front and side on
- The weight stays close to you
- Brace the upper trapezius before pulling
- An incorrect clean that's not powered by the legs is called a muscle clean

- Common mistake is bending the arm before coming into full extension
- Clean with your legs and not your arms
- Review your technique if you experience pain or tenderness around the elbow flexors
- Always end up with a good insert and racking position
- Never stay straight while dropping the weight and letting the weight jerk on the shoulders
- If you're working on your flexibility then you can do hang clean to progress to the dead clean
- There should be no rubbing on the palm of the hand
- The skin is bypassed during the insert

Kettlebell dead clean:

1. Bell placed between the feet
2. Squat
3. Look ahead
4. Hook grip
5. Slight tension between you and the weight
6. Think about pulling the weight to the ceiling
7. Press the heels into the ground
8. Pull the knees back
9. Push the hips forward
10. Keep the arm extended for as long as possible
11. Use the power from the legs
12. Don't curl the weight
13. Let the bell travel up further
14. Open up
15. Hand insert
16. Let the bell come around the fist and not over
17. Come into full racking position
18. Loose grip
19. Let the weight drop
20. Pull back and out
21. Hook grip

22. Reduce velocity with the legs
23. Gently place the weight dead on the ground
24. Repeat

Look ahead

No need to look at the kettlebell, maintain good form and alignment, keep your sight ahead, not down.

Extended elbow

Pull with legs, not with the elbow flexors, this means you keep the elbow extended for as long as is required to generate the right amount of power with the legs.

Accelerated pull

The pulling speed needs to increase, accelerate and generate enough power to make the weight float.

Hips low; shoulders high

This is not a hip hinge, it's a squat, drop you hips low and keep your shoulders high.

Float, open + insert

Make the weight float, i.e. get it to the point where it's weightless, then open the hand, let the bell come around, and insert the hand into the window.

Full racking position

End up in full racking position, even if your next rep is another dead clean, complete the full movement and don't get sloppy.

Controlled landing

Don't let the bell just crash on the floor, control the descent and gently put the kettlebell back dead on the ground.

Drop + pull-out

Let the kettlebell drop back down, pull the hand back out, transition back into hook grip.

Drop + pull back

While the bell drops, pull the elbow back, keeping it where it is means that the bell will move away from the body, you want a direct path back down.

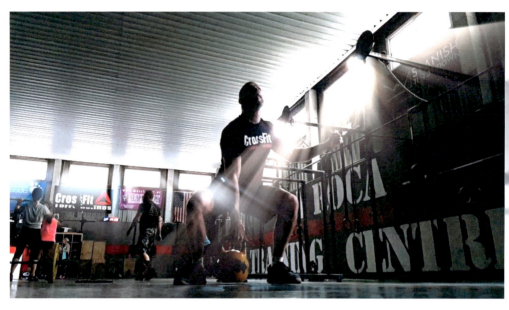
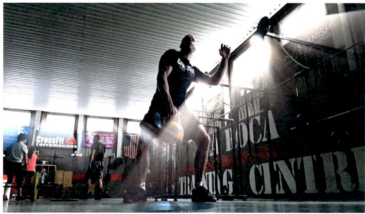

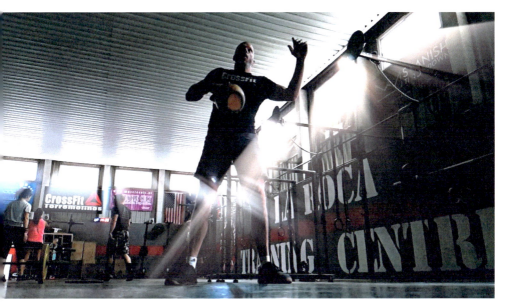
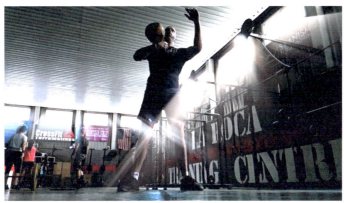
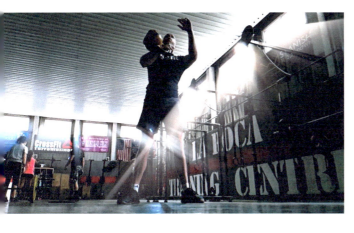

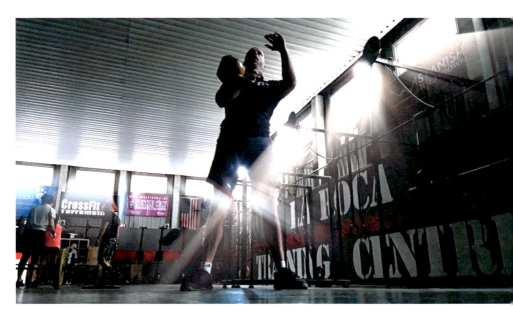
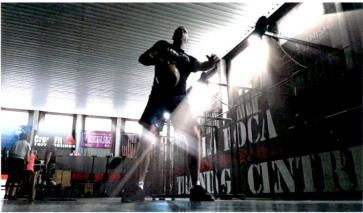
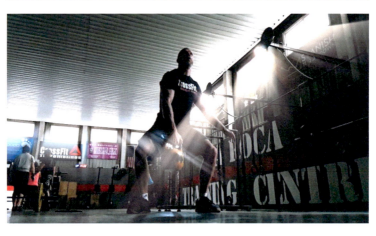

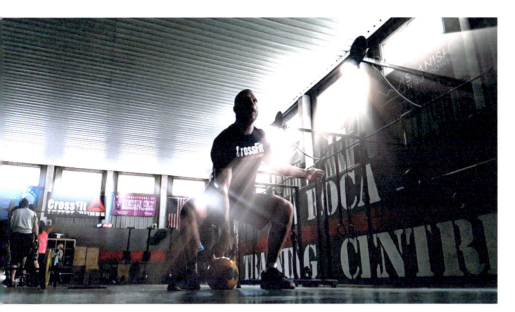

Common mistakes

Swinging

The kettlebell should go up and down in one straight path, the kettlebell should not move away from the body, when it's away from the body and then needs to land between the feet, it will turn into a swing.

Curling

This is a clean, not a curl, a clean is always powered by the lower-body, hence, no bicep curling, no matter how light the weight is. Bicep curling will not only promote bad technique, but also bring along a host of other issues, like tendon injury etc.

Light weight

Using a weight too light promotes bad technique, the weight needs to provide adequate resistance to be able to give the legs the resistance they need to become explosive and have good technique.

Tight grip

Employ a loose hook grip, transition into racking grip, back into hook grip, never hold the kettlebell handle tight.

Task

Your eleventh task is to complete as per below.

Train your dead clean and work your way up over time:

1. 12kg/26.4lbs
2. 16kg/35.2lbs
3. 20kg/44lbs

Duration and sets:

- 2 reps each side
  1 set and 10 seconds rest
  Repeat 4 times

- 4 reps each side
  1 set and 15 seconds rest
  Repeat 4 times

- 6 reps each side
  1 set and 20 seconds rest
  Repeat 4 times

Program each progression until you feel comfortable. For example, the first week you might do 3 days of 12kg and 2 reps. The next week you increase the reps to 4 and so on. At the end you move up in weight for the next 3 weeks until you've completed 20kgs.

Submission

You can film your dead clean for feedback. Submit your video in any way possible. See chapter on How to submit your assessment.

Day 12 Kettlebell swing clean

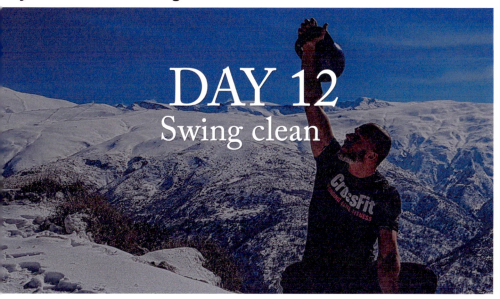

On day 12 you will learn the most common version of the kettlebell clean, the swing clean. The swing clean clean is the most common clean used for clean and press, clean and jerk, etc. I will demonstrate that you can swing clean with a squat, hip hinge, and pendulum so that you can create the clean that works and feels good for you.

Dot points:

- The same concept as with the dead clean applies and you want to drive that weight up
- Use the legs to clean and at the top open up to perform a hand insert
- You can clean with; Hip hinge; Squat; Pendulum
- Keep the weight close to you
- A good drill is the towel drill to practice elbow to body proximity
- If the towel falls then your elbow was not in the right place

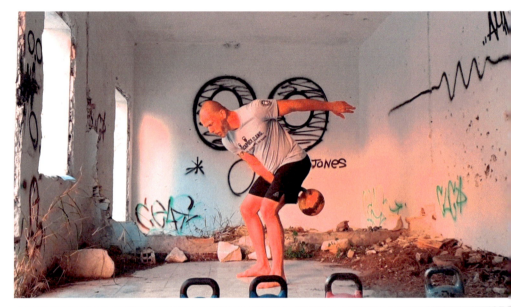
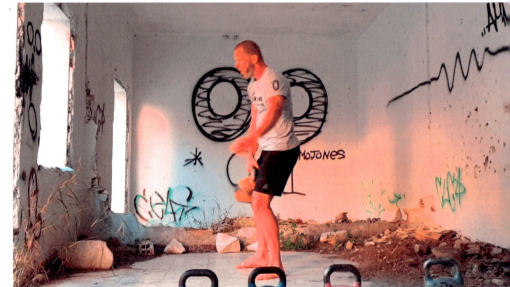

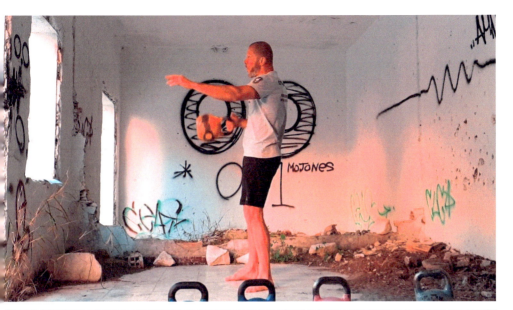

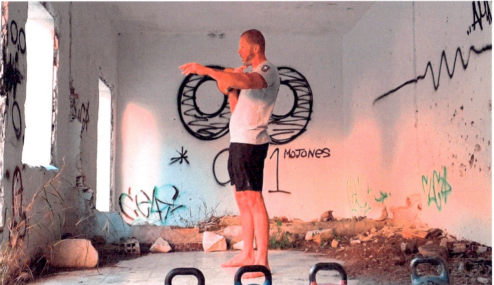

Task

Your twelfth task is to complete as per below.

Train your swing clean and work your way up over time:

1. 8kg/17.6lbs
2. 12kg/26.4lbs
3. 16kg/35.2lbs

Duration and sets:

- 4 reps each side
  1 set and 10 seconds rest
  Repeat 4 times

- 6 reps each side
  1 set and 20 seconds rest
  Repeat 4 times

- 8 reps each side
  1 set and 30 seconds rest
  Repeat 4 times

Program each progression until you feel comfortable. For example, the first week you might do 3 days of 8kg and 4 reps. The next week you increase the reps to 6 and so on. At the end you move up in weight for the next 3 weeks until you've completed 16kgs. Perform double kettlebells if you want to take it a step further. 4 reps each side would just become 4 reps one time.

Submission

You can film your swing clean for feedback. Submit your video in any way possible. See chapter on How to submit your assessment.

Day 13 Kettlebell racking

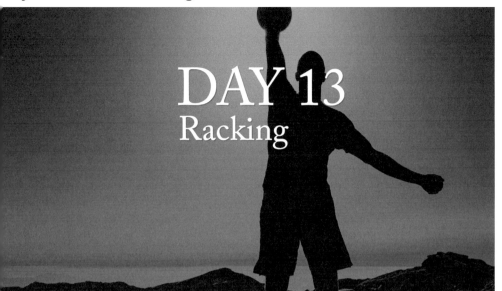

On day 13 you will learn how to rack a kettlebell properly and with the least amount of effort. Racking is what happens after the clean or after bring the kettlebell down from overhead. Racking may seem unimportant and simple, but it's not, it's super important to get your racking right and I will explain why and show you how to get your rack right. I will also cover racking for females.

Dot points:

- Kettlebell racking happens after you clean a kettlebell
- The rack can be a resting or transitional position
- A bad racking position can burn out the shoulders or affect the forearm
- With a transitional rack your elbow should be tucked/pulled into your obliques/ribs
- Use your latissimus dorsi to pull the elbow/arm in
- Rest the bell on the biceps and forearm
- A little bit of space at the bottom of the elbow is ok for a transitional rack
- For jerking or push pressing you want to rest the elbow on the ilium to transfer power
- For resting you want to rest the elbow on the ilium
- During sport/endurance/high volume reps you want to use a good rack to be able to rest with the bell up
- A disconnected arm means shoulder flexion which means additional and unnecessary work

- Let the weight rest on your skeletal system and not your muscular system
- Although it might look like it's bad for the lumbar there is actually no movement in the lumbar
- All range is created through hip hyper extension and extension plus flexion in the thoracic
- A good rack requires flexibility in the hips and thoracic
- Squeeze the gluteus maximus to pull the top of the pelvis back
- Let the top of the femur come slightly forward
- Getting better range in the hip flexors takes time
- Hip hyper extension and crunch
- A rounded back is not a problem because we're not pressing
- You want to rack with just enough contraction to obtain a good posture
- The weight naturally wants to fall away from the body which requires work to pull in
- Make space to let the weight rest on/above the legs
- The cradle rack is an option for females with larger breasts
- The rack is a position you need to learn properly

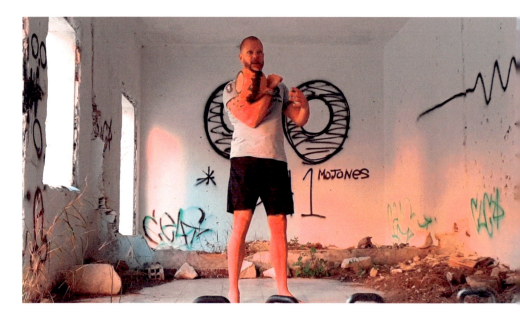

Task

Your thirteenth task is to complete as per below.

Drill your racking and work your way up over time:

1. 8kg/17.6lbs
2. 12kg/26.4lbs
3. 16kg/35.2lbs

Duration and sets:

- 15s each side
  *1 set and 30 seconds rest
  Repeat 4 times*

- 30s each side
  *1 set and 45 seconds rest
  Repeat 4 times*

- 45s each side
  *1 set and 60 seconds rest
  Repeat 4 times*

- 60s each side
  *1 side and 30 seconds rest
  Repeat 4 times*

Program each progression until you feel comfortable. For example, the first week you might do 3 days of 8kg and 15s work. The next week you increase the time under the rack to 30s and so on. At the end you move up in weight for the next 4 weeks until you've completed double 16kgs. Perform double kettlebells if you want to take it a step further. 15s each side would just become 15s one time.

Submission

You can film your racking for feedback. Submit your video in any way possible. See chapter on How to submit your assessment.

Day 14 Kettlebell pressing

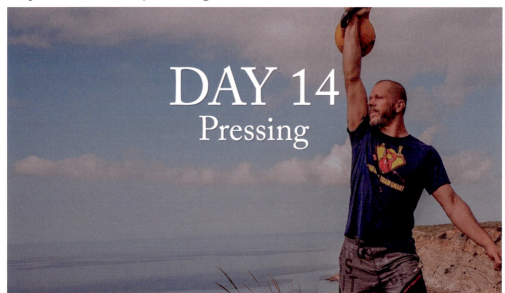

On day 14 you will learn how to press a kettlebell overhead. Before pressing you need to clean and rack, hence the reason I've covered the clean and rack first. I will demonstrate and string all three things together, cleaning, racking, and pressing. With all 3 of these under your belt you can already being to create little full body workouts for yourself like, clean, rack, squat, and press.

Dot points:

- Before you can press you will need to clean and rack
- I'm covering the overhead press but there is also the chest press which is not covered
- Before you press create tension and lock everything out so not to lose power during the press
- Tension and locking out creates a stable base to press from but also recruits more muscles
- Protect your lower back through gluteus maximus contraction (and hamstrings)
- As the bell comes overhead you're moving underneath it
- You want to end up directly under the kettlebell
- It's ok to work on overhead range with a light weight
- The triceps lock out the elbow
- Keep the shoulder safe through lat engagement and pulling the scapulae slightly down
- Once overhead let the weight rest on the skeletal system but keep pressing up

- Obtain a good overhead lockout on each rep
- Work on full range for mobility and flexibility
- Full range means longer under tension which is good for strength
- Keep the elbow under the weight during the press

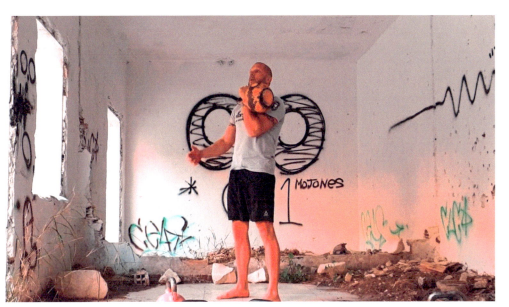

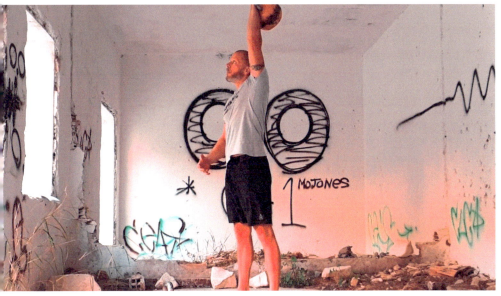

Task

Your fourteenth task is to complete as per below.

Train your press and work your way up over time:

1. 8kg/17.6lbs
2. 12kg/26.4lbs
3. 16kg/35.2lbs

Duration and sets:

- 4 reps each side
  1 set and 10 seconds rest
  Repeat 4 times

- 6 reps each side
  1 set and 15 seconds rest
  Repeat 4 times

- 8 reps each side
  1 set and 20 seconds rest
  Repeat 4 times

Submission

You can film your pressing for feedback. Submit your video in any way possible. See chapter on How to submit your assessment.

Day 15 Kettlebell rowing

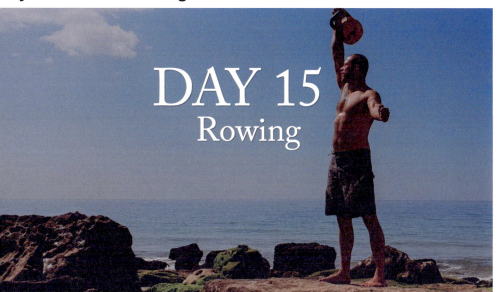

On day 15 you will learn how to perform the bent-over row which is a must do exercise to work the muscles in the back. Rowing is great to work the rear delts but also works lots of other muscles in the back including the all important erector spinae muscle groups.

Dot points:

- The row as demonstrated targets the rear delts but other muscles of the back are involved
- You can row while supporting the torso or without
- Rowing without support challenges the core muscles more
- Rowing with support allows you to isolate and focus on the row more
- Relax the elbow flexors while rowing
- Pull the elbow back into the hip and past
- If the weight starts dead on the ground it's a dead row
- If your hand is coming toward the shoulder you're curling instead of rowing
- Control the movement and get out of it what you're working out for
- Master the movement first and then go high reps and heavier weight
- Nothing but the arms that are working should be moving
- The row demonstrated is the safest in regards to angle between the elbow and ribs

- The bigger the angle between the elbow and ribs the more emphasis will be placed on the middle of the back
- The closer your elbow is to the body the safer it is for beginners
- There are many more ways to perform the kettlebell row

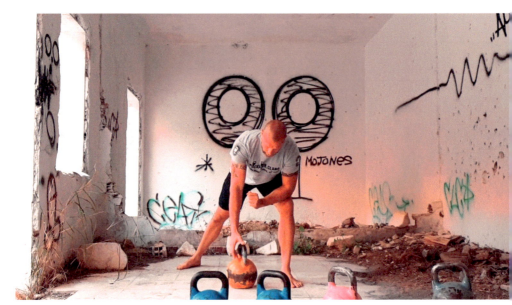

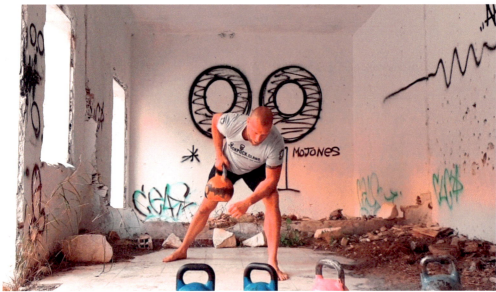

Task

Your fifteenth task is to complete as per below.

Day 16 Kettlebell American swing

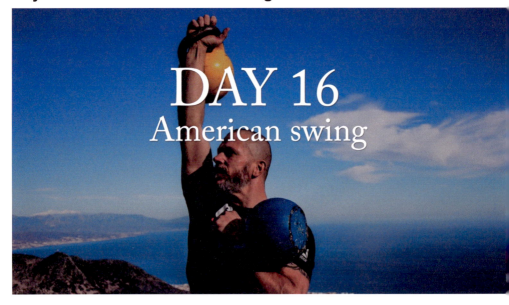

On day 16 you will learn how to perform the American swing which is the most popular version of the swing in CrossFit. The objective and height of this swing is completely different to the previous versions of the swing that I covered.

Dot points:

- The American swing is a swing that does involve a shoulder raise
- This version of the swing is created by CrossFit
- Before you do this exercise you need to check if you can safely/easily bring your arms above your head with a close grip
- The American swing is great if you want to work your shoulders and legs at the same time
- The swing can be performed with a squat, hip hinge, or pendulum

The American swing:

- Perform a swing
- Follow through with a shoulder raise
- Lock the arms out overhead
- Let the bell drop back with slightly bent arms to keep the drop closer
- Guide into the backswing and repeat

You can also replace the raise with a press out and treat this as a double arm snatch.

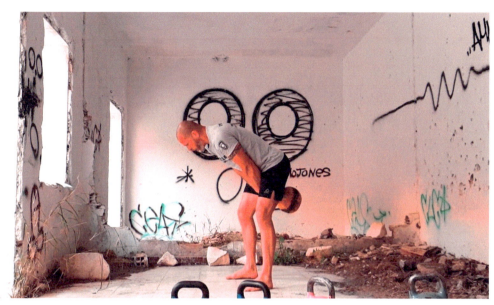

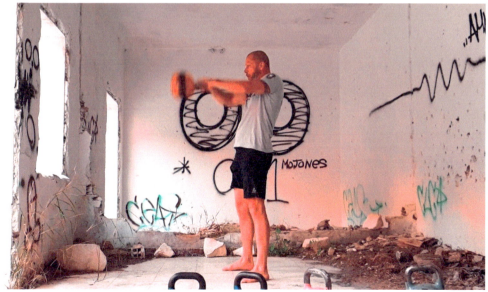

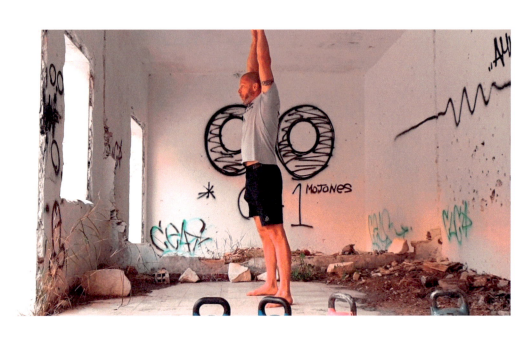

Day 17 Double kettlebell dead swing clean

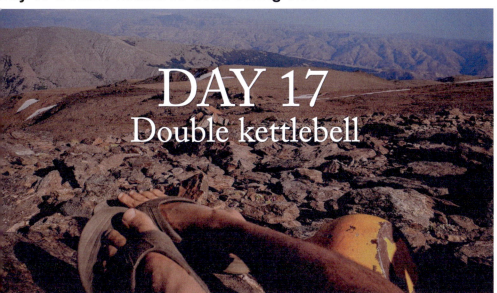

On day 17 you will learn how to clean double kettlebells to lay a basic foundation to start working with double kettlebells when you've mastered all previous steps. However, double kettlebell sounds complex and advanced, but in some cases I've found that people actually get the technique quicker when working with two bells, hence, I like to include it in this course to see if it works for you.

Dot points:

- Double kettlebell work is great to add additional weight to your workout
- Some double bell exercises are but not limited to; front squat; shoulder press; swing; etc.
- How the arm is rotated (where the thumb points) has an effect on the clean
- The effect it has is not covered but you should know that there is so much more to learn about the clean for efficiency
- Safety racking grip is the grip you should implement with double kettlebells
- There is a free PDF you can download which has over 25+ kettlebell grips including the flat hand and others for double bell
- When working with two kettlebells your legs need to be further apart
- Don't get your fingers caught in between the handles when working with double kettlebells

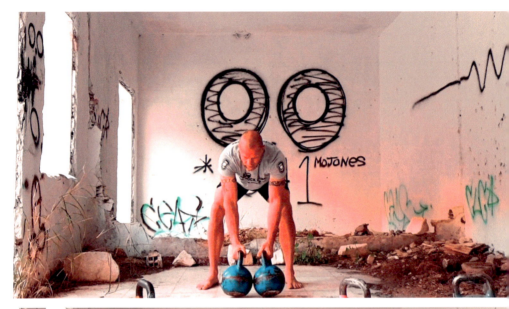
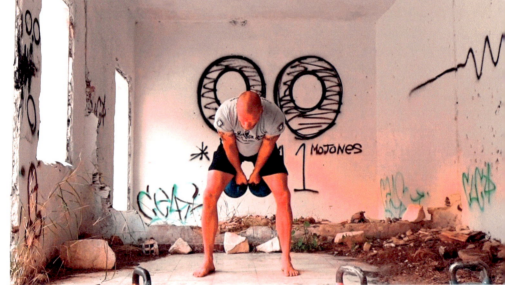

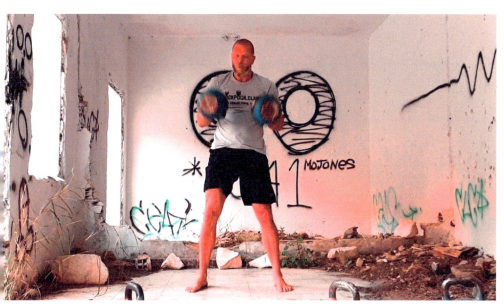
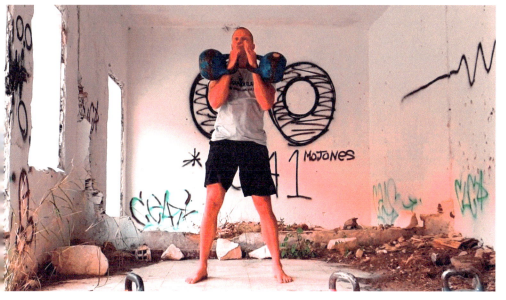

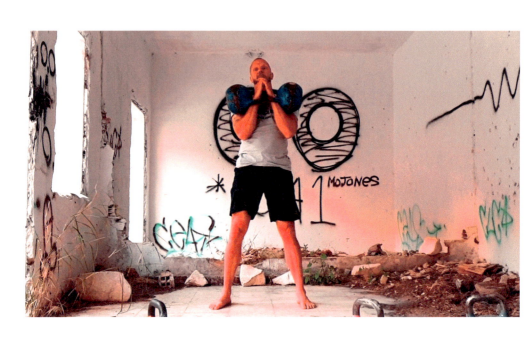

Day 18 Recap and additional kettlebell tips

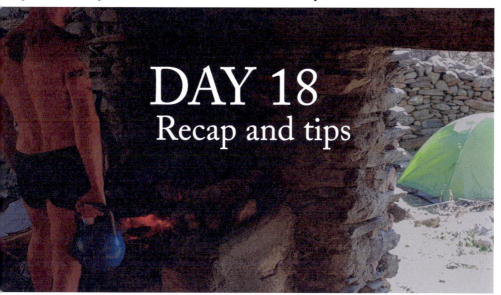

On day 18 I will recap some of the previous days and add additional tips for most of them.

Dot points:

- Warming up and muscle priming are super important
- Mobility work and stretches should become part of your regular training
- Kettlebell grips and assisted clean should be drilled often
- With the dead clean you want to get the power generation right to avoid banging
- If you do come too high you want to come toward and catch the bell
- Don't wait for the bell to bang when it went too high
- This early catch should only be used when working on getting the power
- Don't cast your bell out with the clean to avoid a jolt on the shoulder or lower back
- Move yourself away from the bell to create counter balance
- You need good thoracic and hip mobility to be able to perform this correctly
- Don't follow the kettlebell
- Let the weight drop naturally and guide it back
- Tensing the other arm creates even tension throughout the upper body
- Don't press away from you but up and back to overhead

- If you've progressed with strength and technique you can start looking at pressing away (more advanced)

Day 19 Kettlebell programming and goals

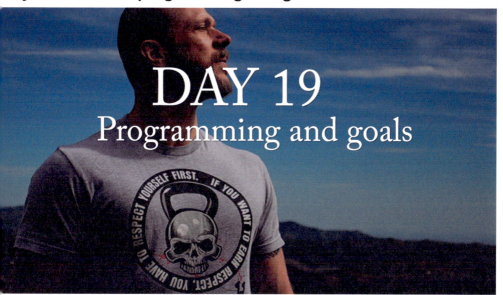

On day 19 I cover some information about basic programming and goals.

Dot points:

- Setting goals in training is important even if those goals are generic training
- Proper programming will help you reach your goals correctly and safely
- Programming involves choosing the right exercises
- Programming for safety involves choosing the right weights and reps
- Identify your goals and write them down
- Figure out how to program to reach those goals
- Training without goals is training for generic fitness
- There is nothing wrong with training for generic fitness
- Find someone to help you reach your goals or do your own research on the topic
- To train for cardiovascular endurance you take lighter weight and work with higher reps
- To train for strength or hypertrophy you go heavier with lower reps and more rest
- To train for flexibility and increased range of motion you program exercises that can challenge your range
- The kettlebell is a weight and can help to reach just about any goal with the right technique and programming behind you

- Due to the design of the kettlebell it is more versatile and optimal for functional movements
- Proper programming is not easy
- To program properly you should learn about muscles and their function
- Think joints not muscles to understand what does what
- Increase weight gradually
- Increase complexity gradually
- Increase rest as you go up with weight
- Control the concentric and eccentric phase and own the movement
- If you're progressing to speed reps then leave the hip hinge deadlift for slow reps for now
- Master the exercise before entering the world of high intensity

TAKE NOTE

The recommendations made in regards to programming are for **beginners**, i.e. assuming you still need to work on strength, coordination, form and technique but still wanting a cardio workout.

Low reps per exercise and muscle groups but performing longer unbroken durations to work on cardio. Once advanced, you can perform longer sets per exercise.

The idea is to increase speed but not to overload muscles and work with bad form and technique, we want to avoid that at all cost. However, once you have mastered an exercise and can identify when form and technique go bad, then it's time to go for longer.

Longer sets are great to work on technique but not under the umbrella of getting is as many reps as possible within the defined amount of time, or getting in a set amount of reps as fast possible. All these types of training are good, but not when you're needing to focus on technique and have other areas to improve upon first.

Day 20 Kettlebell workout

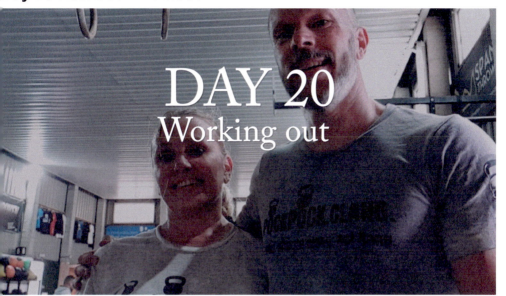

On day 20 you will learn how to string all exercises together and create a few different workouts you can complete.

Workout 1

- Squat dead lift
- Hip hinge dead lift
- Dead swing double arm clean
- Squat
- Press
- Squat thruster (if you feel you're ready)
- Transition to upside down horn grip
- Halo 2 x each side
- Return dead to the ground with a reverse dead swing

Repeat 4 times
Rest 1 minute or include mobility exercises
Work for 20 to 30 minutes.

Notes

The one bell double arm press requires more flexibility than a one arm press. This version of the press is great to work on overhead mobility but you need to progress gently, remember that you can just press half way, next week a bit further, and so on. The double arm press is great to make a heavy weight light enough to press.

If you don't feel comfortable with the transition for the halo grip then add the extra time and relax, put the weight down and pick it up as shown, don't use another complex in the air transition.

Over time you can increase the reps and instead of 1 repetition you can do 2, for example, first 2 weeks you do 1 rep of each exercise, week 3 and 4 you do 2 reps of each exercise, week 5 and 6 you do 3 reps of each exercise and so on till about 6 to 8 reps exercise. You can also increase duration of the workout.

Workout 2

This workout is slightly more advanced than the first one and is programmed more for cardio and endurance.

- One arm swing
- One arm clean
- One arm strict press

Switch at will.

Work for 5 or 10 minutes
Rest in rack

Notes

Rest or reduce weight if you can no longer perform a strict press. Chose your weight carefully at the start.

Create your own workout

Put your own workout together with the exercises you've learned. Feel free to post a copy of your workout with the goals, weight, reps, rest, etc.

I have put together many other beginners workouts for you which you can view on YouTube.

8-minute kettlebell workout www.youtube.com/watch?v=Z75BlIc3zlM

Kettlebell Workout WKV 3 Beginner youtu.be/fOnQgLWwqhY

The Basics—Kettlebell Beginner Workout 3 Exercises youtu.be/jkXtJEF7GuQ

Beginner Workout For Total Body WKV1 youtu.be/rZ_pSdcQIIU

Simple Kettlebell Workout 10 min. Kettlebell youtu.be/ygmFTFdfke8

8 Minute Kettlebell Workout youtu.be/e0q4kHO4okU

Kettlebell Strength Workout - THE BIG FOUR youtu.be/mUyu6haFo8c

This last one is a bit more advanced but still contains all the exercises you've learned in this book but it's performed with two kettlebells. You can perform this with one kettlebell and just double the rounds.

Day 21 Common kettlebell injuries and annoyances

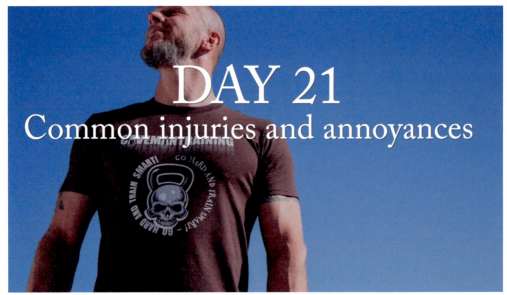

On day 21 you will learn how to avoid common injuries and annoyances with kettlebell training.

Dot points:

- The broken wrist grip is where you don't obtain a good hand insert
- Pressing with a broken wrist grip affects the wrists and can cause injury or pain
- Focus on the assisted clean drill
- Don't work with a broken wrist grip even if the weight is light
- Take your time to get the hand insert right if you intend to train with kettlebells for a long time
- Lower back problems are common with the kettlebell because of the dynamic movements
- The kettlebell is not at fault and neither are the exercises
- The kettlebell requires respect and dedication
- Don't throw the kettlebell out and follow it
- Don't lift with the back but use the muscles intended
- Go back to MMC and muscle priming if back aches occur
- Look at programming when aches occur
- Don't hold the kettlebell too tight or let it flip over the fist

- Kettlebell training does not need to hurt if you invest the time
- Maintain the calluses on your hands
- Work on technique and do not wear gloves
- If you have blisters you need to look at your technique or programming
- Friction occurs in the hand when you don't open up during the clean or the kettlebell bobs during swinging
- The handle does not need to rub when moving directly from hook grip into the 45 degree angle
- Bypass your skin during the clean and insert
- The kettlebell should remain a direct extension of your arm during the swing
- In the beginning you can't avoid mild bruising on your forearm as there has never been a weight resting on it before
- Additional pressure on the forearm can be created by too much wrist flexion
- Grabbing the handle in the middle will result in the middle of the bell providing unnecessary pressure on the forearm

VOUCHER CODES

To get the course on Udemy you can directly access the following link and get 50% off.

https://www.udemy.com/kettlebell-training-for-beginners/?couponCode=CT35I1VZ09

CT35I1VZ09

To get 50% discount on the kettlebell training app that allows you to cast the videos to your TV or watch on your phone email me on me@tacofleur.com with the subject "Voucher code for kb app from Amazon book" and include the following verification code in the body "291VM9OC". I will reply to your email and send you a unique voucher code with detailed instructions to get 50% off on the app. The way Google is setup I can't include the codes in the book.

Details of the app here

https://play.google.com/store/apps/details?id=com.cavemantraining.kb.beginners

Ready to move to the next level in your kettlebell training?
Check out the following books by Cavemantraining

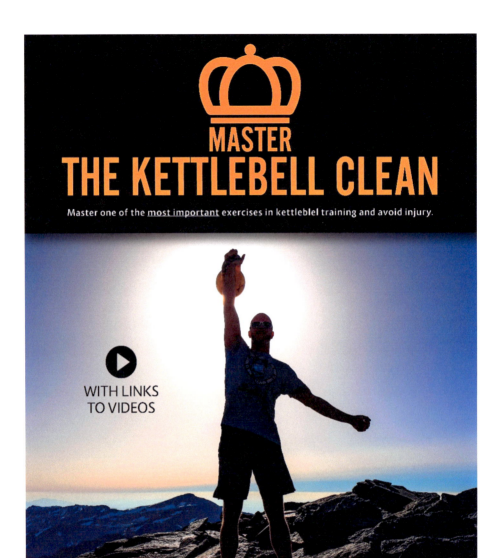

https://amzn.to/2FOJfmy

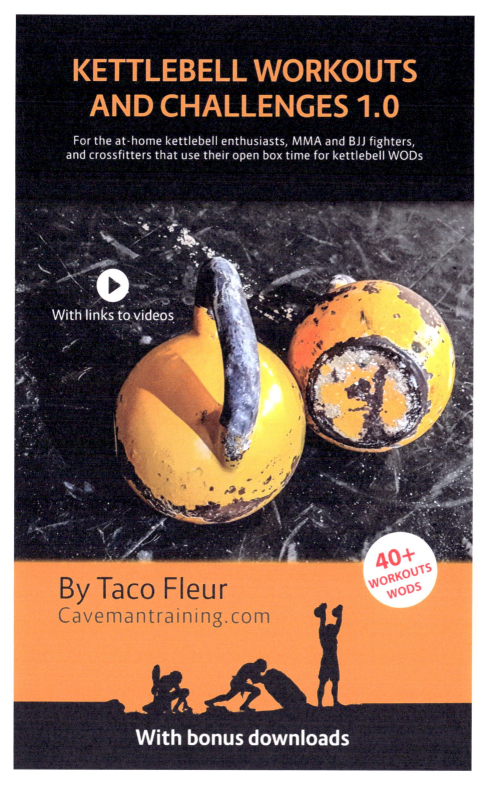

https://amzn.to/2FHgfwN

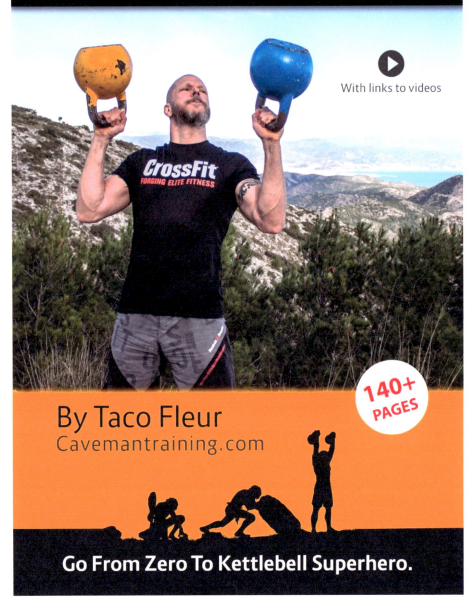

https://amzn.to/2TQYvnC

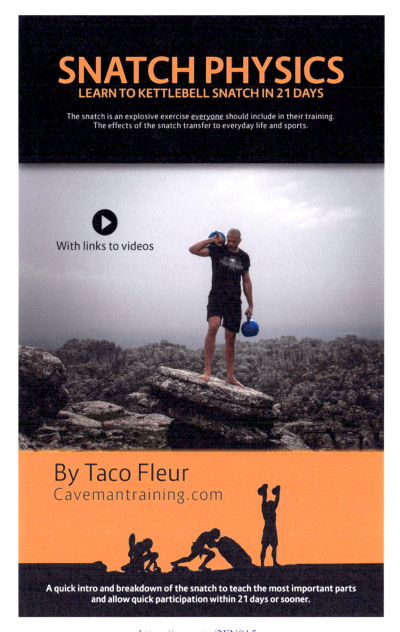

https://amzn.to/2FN015v

All books can be found here on Amazon amzn.to/2FUyaQX or on www.cavemantraining.com/shop

I hope you enjoyed this book and I hope to see more of you on your kettlebell journey, come and join me on Facebook and say hi:

The biggest kettlebell training group on Facebook www.facebook.com/groups/KettlebellTraining

Kettlebell workouts on Facebook www.facebook.com/groups/kettlebell.workout

Kettlebell training group on Reddit www.reddit.com/r/kettlebell_training

Hundreds of videos on YouTube youtube.com/Cavemantraining

Me on Instagram instagram.com/realcavemantraining/

If you can find a couple of seconds to rate the book on Amazon I would really appreciate it.

Thanks

Taco Fleur

Printed in France by Amazon
Brétigny-sur-Orge, FR